Recycling Me

Back on the Bike

By

Kate Bosley

To my husband John,

My children Charlotte, Hannah,

Josh and Sarah,

My Mum and Dad, Janet and Bernard,

My friend Karen,

And all who helped me to recover

And to write this book.

CONTENTS

PREFACE

It is shaky, to say the least, that I expect people to read a book about the dramatic experience that I have gone through and then written about. It is shaky for two good reasons. The first is that my memory is significantly challenged and I remember little of the past. I have had to speak to my husband and children to explain to me what happened and then I have had to write it down later. It is clear from what they told me that I suffered a major head injury, was in a coma for two weeks and was expected to die by both the medics and my family. I have only been able to document what happened because I have been told their version of events truthfully and with some degree of patience, as I have needed them to repeat it several times.

The second reason is the dyslexia I have always suffered from. I can't believe many dyslexics want to write things down and expect others to read it. I know that under normal circumstances I wouldn't have wanted to, but over the last year enough people have said "Write it down" that I began to think I am going to give it go - even though I know I will struggle to write it down in a way that is interesting to read, despite having a computer and an offer of help.

Tell me what you think!

So before I tell the story of our event I think it might be useful to know a little bit about me - who I am, or should I say who I was. I won't go on too much, I promise. I will also briefly say a bit about my children and my husband John, as they feature strongly in the account. John has been fantastic and in many ways had a worse experience than I did.

CHAPTER ONE – EARLY HISTORY

I was 50 years old and was doing well in life. I was happy in my career and family life. I was a keen cyclist and worked as a chief executive for the local hospice. I trained as a nurse in the 80s - it was my passion but I was a nervous nurse. I cared about doing the right thing. I would have hated doing anything significantly wrong. It scared me but I loved doing it right. When a patient or relative looked relieved I felt great satisfaction. I could make a difference.

I was seeing my boyfriend regularly and had sort of decided that in time we would marry. His parents fostered and I thought he would be a good dad when I saw him with children. This was important to me as I planned a big family. He studied in Sunderland and I trained as a nurse in Leeds. We saw each other regularly and often looked after his brother and sister - his parents had adopted them by then. We used to take his brother aged 7 to his university digs to stay. You weren't allowed anyone to stay, let alone girlfriend and young brother. I loved it and dreamed of a time when I had my own children.

I enjoyed being with young people and after I qualified I took a job in the bone marrow transplant unit. This was new dramatic treatment in the 1980s although I know it is done more frequently now. The unit cared for adults and children and was extremely valuable experience for me. We had to wear theatre clothes. We would scrub up especially clean and perform total care for our patients, which included cooking meals and cleaning the room as well as giving blood and drugs intravenously. It gave me good experience in long term and total support. The unit had two beds and patients took weeks to recover well enough to be discharged. We lost several patients and I found it a struggle coming to terms with their deaths. It was particularly difficult when you felt that you had known them so long and cared for them and their families closely.

It made me think about life more deeply than others my age who I was in contact with. I wanted to do things with my life and enjoy it as much as I could. Having goals helped me achieve things that I wouldn't have achieved otherwise.

John and I married in 1982. I was still doing general nursing but wanted to become a children's nurse. I began my paediatric training, specialising as a nurse for sick children at Great Ormond Street Hospital in London. John was interested in special needs teaching. So we were both moving forward in our chosen careers.

Great Ormond Street taught me lots. Once qualified, I worked in the Oncology ward. I wondered why such terrible things could happen to such lovely young children. A child dying didn't and still doesn't feel right. I loved being with them, though. I also enjoyed supporting parents and couldn't believe how brave they all were. There are no training courses to help people cope with that experience. It made me very nervous when I became pregnant. What if it happened to us? I nursed and respected lots of lovely children who died. This made me feel different when I had my own - I was much more nervous than normal.

John was enjoying working with people with learning difficulties. He worked in a day unit for adults with special needs. I think he recognised that he had the possibility of developing his career - a career doing something he really enjoyed - and he progressed from the day care unit to the local special school where he started his career as a teacher, having qualified whilst I was at Great Ormond Street.

We had been married for a short time when we decided that we wanted children but I was unsure as to the best way forward. I decided to leave Great Ormond Street and work near our Newbury home where John was working. I got a job working for Mencap. I worked in a newly renovated house for clients with learning difficulties. It was great fun. Working closely alongside those with massive challenges changed my thinking. Their challenges were different from what I was used to and they coped by making the best of it. They taught me a great deal and I enjoyed my time with them.

So the job was different and challenging but I felt that I understood what it was like to have a learning disability. Society didn't understand. It amazed me how challenged people could be and how difficult life could be for them. Little did I know that I would become disabled later in life. Although I am sure I made a difference to people I know now that I didn't fully understand the complex feelings you can have when it happens to you.

John moved on to become a teacher. He seemed to like it and we both felt babies might happen.

CHAPTER TWO- BECOMING PARENTS

I became pregnant straight away. We argued about names but eventually agreed on Charlotte for a girl and Thomas if it was a boy. Charlotte was born in Reading and it wasn't easy. I won't bore you with details as this book isn't about the challenges of labour but it wasn't a great experience and John had a lot to cope with. I had to go to theatre a couple of times.

Charlotte was a demanding baby - you knew you had her. I was experienced with sick babies but I found her difficult. She seemed to test you. However she was lovely and we both enjoyed being parents enormously. John was teaching and was out all day and I stayed at home, met friends who had babies the same age as Charlotte, and generally enjoyed being with her. We still lived in Newbury in a small modern three bedroomed house. We eventually decided a bigger home was important and the stresses of selling and buying a house started. We were successful and moved across town.

Parenthood was fun as well as hard work and we soon wanted another baby. In my mind I would have liked to have delivered normally without fuss. It's what most people do, isn't it? Charlotte was only 22 months old when my second baby arrived. We decided not to find out what sex she was before giving birth. Hannah was born more normally than the others but it wasn't a particularly easy delivery and there was a problem with her breathing. I had tried NCT classes the second time around to see if this would help me deliver well. A friend who also took the classes knew someone who had had a cot death in the last year. The local cot death society lent people apnea monitors at no charge. They strapped onto the baby and alarmed when the baby stopped breathing and for peace of mind we had one. Hannah's alarmed all the time. When you got to her she was breathing but appeared to be taking a gasp. We took into account that the alarm may have shocked her into breathing again. We continued with this way of caring for her- getting up several times a night and dealing with it throughout the day when she slept. However it did mean that we were completely at ease. If there was silence in her room she was breathing. It was and still is extremely unusual for people to monitor their babies. I knew people thought I was an over-anxious mother but my nursing career made me worry more than others and I wanted to feel as safe as possible and enjoy the babies as much as I could. I loved two children.

I knew my children were lucky (although they might say differently now). I was concerned about children who didn't have parents and wondered whether there was anything we could do to help those children. We had enquired about fostering prior to Hannah's birth but were told that we couldn't foster while I was pregnant. It was decided that we could reapply later when the baby was settled.

John (as you know) was teaching children with learning difficulties. He came in from work one day and said that there was a child in his class who needed fostering urgently. It seemed that he had been in foster care for most of his life but wasn't lucky enough to find foster parents that suited him. John's experience of working with people with learning difficulties and my passion for helping people with problems made us feel there was a good chance we could do it. It was an extremely unusual situation but eventually we were successful in our application and J G, who was 16 years old, came to live with us. He was great with the babies and seemed to enjoy being with them. He was at school in the daytime, which meant I had time with the babies. We felt a lot of people didn't understand why we did it. I have to say I think it has been a positive experience. He is still part of my life and has had a huge impact on me. It is a different love from the love I have for my own children but it is a special love. I still see him weekly.

In many ways we all benefited from fostering J G. My children have grown up understanding special needs. They take into account that all people are different but all are valuable in their own unique way. Sarah, my youngest daughter, who actually wasn't born when we fostered J G, was talking on the phone to him yesterday. The skills she used were quite advanced and I'm proud of her, proud of all my children. In so many ways they have benefited. Of course sharing your parent also asks a lot of a child. It wasn't always easy! We carried on fostering J G for three years until his 19th birthday. (It was the plan when he arrived, as you leave fostering when you're 19 if you have a learning disability.)

I enjoyed life with J G and the two children and as things started to get easier we decided to have another baby. I became pregnant for the third time. Looking back I think it may have been a little insane to have three so close together.

John decided to move schools to further his career. He applied for a teaching job in Maidstone, Kent, which was very near where my parents lived. When he secured the job we were delighted. I was heavily pregnant at the time and so we moved to Maidstone just weeks before I had the baby, probably causing chaos for the midwives and GP in our new area. Again the delivery was challenging. Josh was born with a large blue/grey mark on his leg. It was filled with blood vessels and was about the size of a golf ball on a newborn baby's leg. I wasn't sure what it was and hadn't seen anything like it in my nursing career. I was most concerned that it could be malignant but had to wait the rest of the night and half the next day to see the doctor. He told me it was a birthmark and probably would not disappear completely, although it was extremely unlikely to be harmful to his life. I was very pleased with this diagnosis as I had feared something worse. It's interesting, though, because John wasn't particularly reassured. He had expected to be told that the mark would fade and disappear in time. We now had to explain to our child to be careful with the mark as it could bleed heavily and we were worried that he might grow up with negative feelings that a quarter of his leg looked different. But Josh just got on with it and hasn't been bothered at all. As I write this it's his birthday. Twenty-three years ago we were worried but now it's not a problem to me and I don't think it's a problem to Josh. It made me realise that diagnoses can mean different things to different people. As a nurse you need to find out what it means to a particular individual and not make assumptions about what they might be feeling.

We moved in Maidstone a few times, in the end buying a bungalow which needed a lot of renovation but which would be a fantastic family home as the children grew older. I recognised that we could be happy living there for a long time as our children grew.

J G moved on when he became 19. When he left I was devastated - I missed him enormously but was helped by being so busy. We didn't receive any support from social services but were expected to get on with it. I had found J G a challenge but no more than the other children. Charlotte was a particular challenge. She hated being controlled by adults and it was clear that she wanted to grow up. She knew what she wanted even as a young child.

I remember when she was two years old we had put her into bed. We heard movement but left her to settle. She clearly didn't want to go to bed but eventually it became quiet. Later on, when we opened the door leading to our stairs, we found her, fast asleep on the stairs, fully dressed. She was wearing a swimming hat, goggles and a swimming costume, all over her nappy. She was so funny!

Hannah was calmer - she seemed to sit beside Charlotte and watch her. However when she did join in she was very able. For example they both entered a painting competition at the local Early Learning Centre. My main focus was Charlotte because she was four and learning to draw. She coloured in the Greek pot very well. I let Hannah join in just to keep her occupied - after all she was only two. The paintings were pinned on the wall of the shop and every week I would check they were still there and how good Charlotte's was compared with others. To be honest I wasn't that surprised when I received a phone call saying my daughter had won and we were to visit the shop to receive a prize voucher. It was only when we went to collect the prize that I realised Charlotte hadn't won. It was of course Hannah who had impressed the judges with her painting. She was only two!

We had bought Charlotte a Brio train set because we both felt it was important that girls had the same opportunity as boys to grow and develop and didn't feel that you should be biased about what they were allowed to play with. However the toy wasn't well valued by either Charlotte or Hannah. It stayed in the back of my cupboard in its box. I was clearing up one day and Josh found it. I hadn't got it out for him to play with because I thought he was too young. However it was an instant success and he took it with him wherever we went. He made fantastically complicated tracks and at one point the set went to the child-minder's house every time Josh went. Sheila had two boys and they also had Brio. However it wasn't Josh's and he loved his set.

CHAPTER THREE – CAREER AND FAMILY

By now I had gone back to work at the local hospital and was on the bank. This meant I was called in whenever they were really short staffed, which was fairly frequently. I worked on the children's ward but had become very interested in the care of people dying. One of my patients was a young boy with a terminal diagnosis, whose pain was difficult to control. This led me to start reading about hospice care. At that time hospice care wasn't well recognized, especially care for children. The more I read about it the more I realised that alternative support was available. In fact a hospice had recently opened in Maidstone.

One day I was reading a local newspaper and saw that there was a vacancy for a Hospice Nurse. It was clear that it was for adults only but I wondered if I could join the bank of nurses at the hospice while also remaining at the hospital. At the time I didn't want permanent work but joining the bank seemed a good idea. I could learn about pain control and if necessary could use the expertise to support young people back at the hospital. I was rather nervous about applying as I hadn't nursed adults for a while. I was interviewed by the matron and I remember that she used to take her dog, a large black Labrador, to work. He was part of the interview panel, staring at me when I was answering questions. I wondered if he was asked about my suitability for the post. I got the job and started soon after.

I loved it and knew from my very first night that my career was going to change. I loved having the time to give excellent care for both the patients and the relatives. I found it so exciting and rewarding to have the time to give each patient the quality of care that you would wish for yourself or a close family member. I knew during that first shift that it was going to be something that I was going to be involved with for a long time. Symptoms were looked at and the doctor would prescribe appropriate medication with an approach quite different from what I was used to. Patients were not only helped by medication but, together with their families, were offered psychological support by skilled staff. The social worker, too, ensured that they were helped with social problems. The families fully appreciated the service we offered.

Only a few weeks after starting bank work at the hospice I was offered a permanent job. This was to prove a major career decision for me.

My job at the hospice suited me in every way. On a practical level I needed less childcare as the hospice shifts tended to be longer. I had a very experienced child-minder called Sheila and by now Charlotte was at school, followed quickly by Hannah.

As well as fitting in with family life the job also satisfied me. I loved my two long shifts per week and soon developed important skills. I received lots of comments from patients and their families saying I had made a difference. I had the odd written comment sent to thank me. My colleagues also did and I knew that I was in a very good team that made a significant impact. Because John was a teacher he had the weekends off. I liked working at the weekend as child-care was no problem, although it did mean that John didn't have rest days. He was either working or delivering child-care by himself. He was enjoying teaching and became the deputy head of a special school.

Having three children was great fun but obviously hard work. We wanted four children but found three hard enough and decided to wait until Josh was at school before considering another baby.

I remember when Josh was about to start school he appeared worried about it. 'What's the matter, Josh?' I asked. 'I thought you were excited about school.' He told me he wanted to go but he was worried that I would be lonely and bored on the days I wasn't working if he was at school. He was genuinely relieved when I told him I would be OK. I promised him, at his request, that if I was bored at home I would collect him from school.

With Josh at school I was able to work a few extra shifts and I enjoyed this. My parents had bought a holiday home in France and we stayed with them a few times. We also borrowed a caravan and enjoyed taking that to France too. We liked cycling and had some bikes with children's seats on the back. I remember us going for a ride - John had two children on his bike, one on the cross bar and one on the back, while I had Charlotte on my bike. We used to ride on the cycle paths near the coast around Bordeaux and it was great fun. We would take the caravan away nearly every year and in time of course the children had their own bikes.

Eventually we decided to have another child. We told the others quite soon after we knew. They were all excited but Charlotte was really keen and quite quickly mentioned what she would think when she saw the baby being born. I explained that children didn't see the birth but visited the hospital afterwards. She was outraged that she couldn't see the birth. I said I would enquire whether it was possible. My midwife said it was unusual but suggested that I showed them a video of births. It was likely that the video would be enough. The video portrayed had five different births. One was a water birth which I was sure wouldn't be suitable for me because of my previous problems giving birth.

We knew we were having a girl and so we looked forward to it. We decided to let the children choose the name. Charlotte took the lead, persuading the others to choose Sarah. I was advised that we would need a second adult at the birth to care for the children should it be lengthy or difficult. So one night in January I went into labour. Josh aged 6 had seen the video and decided that he would prefer to stay at a friend's house. We took him there and collected the girls. To make things complicated it was a night labour and the girls had to stay awake all night. I remember they were mainly bored and tired. I kept going for a walk and at one point started to feel that our plans were not going to work out. The girls were shattered, nothing was happening and they were going to have to go home. I knew they were then likely to miss the birth. Hannah wouldn't be pleased but it would be a particular problem for Charlotte.

Then, remarkably, the baby came! I had decided to have a bath and the children went for a little walk with Sheila. Once I was in the water I realised I was going to deliver. Charlotte and Hannah came running in and the baby was born. Of course it was underwater. We hadn't planned or really thought about a water birth and John was slightly concerned. However Charlotte had watched a water birth on the video. She knew what was happening and, aged 10, appeared to reassure every one. She loved it and was the first to handle the baby. In fact the girls bathed her while I was being sewn up and looked after. It's true that I wasn't well and had significant haemorrhaging. The girls were so well looked after at the hospital and they still say being present at Sarah's birth was important to them. Charlotte said a year or so later "Was it being at the birth that caused me to love her like this? Or would I have loved her anyway?" I explained she would have loved her anyway but I am sure that being present was important to the girls.

After Sarah was born I went back to the hospice. I had been made senior and was studying for qualifications in palliative care. Then I became aware that a children's hospice was being built in Sittingbourne. A hospice for children combined my two loves and I was amazed that such an ideal opportunity had presented itself. I applied and got an interview.

When I went for the interview it was still a building site and I remember having to wear a hard helmet. It was promotion for me because I had applied for the Deputy Head of Care post. It was also a full-time job and I would need to change my childcare so that all the children were cared for together. (I had been using someone else to pick the girls up from school.) We decided to have support at home and luckily Sheila was wanting to give up child-minding anyway.

The children's hospice was interesting but quite different from the adult hospice as there was less care of the dying and more respite care. I loved it and felt that my career was moving forward nicely. I found it acceptable to work and have children as long as I didn't have too many boring domestic jobs so I employed a cleaner and a gardener. This worked well and we managed to have weekends away and nice holidays. The baby was parented by the whole family. It was a busy household. I remember, one night, thinking I ought to put Sarah to bed and told Charlotte that was what I was going to do. She said "Don't worry, Mum, she's already down. I did it an hour ago because she was grotty and seemed tired."

I was gaining management experience but realised that I needed still more. After a few years I saw a job as leader of a children's service within an organization that was community based. I wanted to experience the Hospice at Home service and felt it would increase my management experience. I was successful in my application although sad to leave the children's hospice. Again my experience and expertise of management was developed. I enjoyed being in people's own homes and again giving good care. I moved up on the management structure. I valued being a manager and felt that I could make a difference in shaping the service that was offered.

I gained lots of experience and when the post of Clinical Services Manager became available back at the original hospice I applied and got the job. It was obviously an adult service and I missed the children but in every other way it was a perfect job. In time the hospice decided to change the structure and I applied and became the hospice Chief Executive. So I started as a junior nurse and worked my way up to what was clearly a demanding and important job. My children were fantastic, let me focus on the hospice and didn't give me anything to be concerned about. John didn't move up further in his career because we both felt that if the two of us had equally demanding careers this might create challenges for us as a family.

CHAPTER FOUR - LIFE OUTSIDE WORK
MY LOVE OF CYCLING DEVELOPS

Clearly I had a very busy and challenging job and it was important that I developed a hobby where I could relax from the demands of work. So I started cycling. It all happened because I was searching for a sport I could become involved in. Taking part in sport has always been important to me and played a big part in my life even as a child. At school I had once seen a promotional film about orienteering and had become very interested as a result. My parents decided that they wanted to try it too, so as a family we took part in orienteering events quite regularly, often travelling in our caravan to different parts of the country to compete at weekends. We did this frequently until I left home to take up nursing. As it wasn't a hugely popular sport and there was a limited number of competitors I found that I did well and sometimes won. In fact I was Yorkshire champion one year. Within the sport there were different age categories so my parents and brother were also able to compete and enjoyed it as I did. We even travelled to Switzerland to take part in an event. However when I left home to take up nursing my life became very busy and orienteering was almost forgotten. I did try to encourage John to take it up but as the children arrived it wasn't easy for us to do it regularly.

I also enjoyed running and had performed a couple of marathons when Charlotte was little but clearly it was quite difficult to train when you have young children and for many years I didn't really do anything. However as the children grew I became more and more interested in taking up a sport. Charlotte, Hannah and Josh were good at trampolining and I decided to attend an adult class. We had a competition home trampoline in the garden and I thought it would be good for me. However fairly early on I fell badly in an organised class whilst trying a backflip. This caused quite a stir- my left ankle was extremely painful and I was off work and in plaster for a while. My trampolining career was over.

After a while John bought me a gym ticket as a birthday present. He felt basic training would help me remobilise. However it introduced me to spinning. I saw a group finishing a class and thought it looked fun. I knew enough to think that it would involve little weight bearing so it seemed an ideal solution. I went along one Saturday with a work colleague but I was not fit and found the class a challenge. I remember asking the instructor if he thought I should try again. He encouraged me and after a while I found I was becoming more and more passionate about the classes and attended regularly. I persuaded John to give it a go and he too enjoyed it. We started spinning regularly and getting better and better. My work colleague mentioned one day she would like to go to Cuba and had discovered that there was a charity cycle ride across Cuba. We talked about it and decided to apply. I knew I was getting fit spinning but had limited experience cycling. I was bought a hybrid bike and spent some time riding, getting fitter and more confident.

My colleague suggested we joined the local cycling club. It's an interesting club and has rides each weekend for a range of different abilities. We started one weekend and I thought it was amazing as we cycled 30 miles. We went every week, getting fitter and stronger. I was keen to move up to the next class but my colleague wasn't sure. She liked the rather eccentric nature of the cyclists who weren't interested in racing but loved experiencing the world from their bikes. I was keen to move to a faster group and asked John if he wanted to try it. Straightaway he loved it. In 2006 we managed the ride across Cuba despite the fact that the bikes we were given were totally useless. The only way I could change gear was by getting off, picking the chain up and placing it by hand. It was an easy ride but the quality of the bikes and the lack of interesting food made it rather a challenge.

Nonetheless Cuba was amazing to experience and we raised significant money for the hospice we worked at. Also it inspired us both to do something else.

As John worked in a school he could not take any leave outside school holidays but the hospice staff had to take turns to be off in the school holiday. That meant I was sometimes on holiday when John wasn't. I had read about a trip to India and decided that it would be a fantastic achievement. So we applied and again got places. We had better bikes in India and the route was fantastic. We saw the Taj Mahal which is mind-blowingly beautiful and we also saw some tigers out in the wild which was fascinating- an amazing experience (spoilt only a little by a bad stomach bug) and one I remembered later when I thought I might die. I remember being sad that death might happen but pleased I was leaving lovely children, a fantastic husband and that I had done things I had enjoyed and was proud of.

After the India trip we moved into cycle racing. John and I had heard about time trialing and thought we would have a go. Time trials are races on moving, open roads. You set off at minute intervals and you are timed at the end of a set course. My first race wasn't too bad- I was riding at 20 mph over 10 miles. John was faster than me, though, and as we progressed he remained faster at 10 and 25 mile races but I could beat him at 50 and 100 mile ones. We had found a hobby we both loved. We were out most weekends in the summer. We travelled right across England to attend faster courses. It's a strange sport -you don't do a good time if it's windy and it's cancelled if it's wet, so we spent some time travelling to events that didn't happen and we had to leave without a race.

We trained regularly to improve our times. I had gone 'under the hour', which means I had cycled 25 miles in less than 60 minutes. That's pretty fast and although there were better cyclists than me I was rated 10th in the Best All Rounder competition for GB. We're both very proud of our achievements, pleased that we had a good hobby and one that gave me something else to think of on my days off. I think that is very important, especially in the job I had. We had started to employ a cycle coach who was helping me get fitter and I cycled to work (6 miles) and trained 6 days a week for an hour and 20 minutes each day. We had both cycled from Land's End to John O' Groats and I had cycled from London to Nice as well as doing a cols event in France (cycling up many of the mountains in the Alps). Cycling was a massive part of who we were. We loved it. The children were less tolerant of it and felt we were in the midst of some crisis of ageing, but although they would deny it I think they were secretly impressed. Sarah had started to race locally and appeared quite good. When the children said they wanted to go to Disneyland Paris again, I agreed but only if they cycled there. I was joking when I said it and was surprised when they all agreed. We did it and it was again something I am very proud of.

That's one of the things I've learnt about life - it's best to build positive relationships, take positive opportunities and fit in memorable events that can stay with your loved ones forever should anything happen to you. I will never forget arriving at Disneyland knowing we had all cycled there. We actually had one of the best times together we have ever had. Charlotte's and Hannah's boy friends came with us and only Josh was missing. He could not spare the time from work and so he arrived by car and was able to help drive us all home.

So cycling was important to us both. We had made lots of friends who were cyclists and we knew lots of people who raced with us. The support of cyclists has been invaluable to us both over the last year. I wanted to increase my training and felt it would be good to be with others of the same standard. I searched on the internet and found a company that supplied training in Tenerife. The children were young adults and Sarah was skiing with school at half term. It seemed a fantastic opportunity and so we booked two places and couldn't wait.

CHAPTER FIVE – THE DIFFERENT PERSONALITIES OF MY FAMILY

It was in Tenerife that the accident happened. In order to explain the different reactions of my closest family and friends I have decided to describe my relationship with them and a little about their individual characters.

Charlotte was quite a character. She was a challenging baby but grew into a lovely strong child. We didn't over control her as we both felt that we valued her views enough not to boss her around and that if we did she might rebel. She seemed to respond to this. I thought she would row with us and develop a negative response to our interactions if we didn't give her enough freedom. Even as a young child this was the case but as she grew up we allowed her more and more freedom. She was a great singer and I remember her in the school play. I didn't know what she was doing after school but she was often late home and eventually she told me she had a small part in the school play. However when we went to see it we realised she had misled us as she had a main part with a number of solo songs to sing. I know I am her mother and mothers often think such things but she was, in my opinion, fantastic and very funny. I realised she could take this talent forward. I was excited by this, particularly as Charlotte told me how much she had enjoyed the experience. However she had done it once, for the experience, and would never do it again. Ten years later that is still the case.

She had a boyfriend at 17 and went out with him for a year. He was constantly in our house and stayed overnight regularly. I was most upset when their relationship ended. I hadn't noticed him in the house for a few days so I asked

Charlotte where he was and realised straightaway that she was distressed. It was clearly over.

Charlotte didn't really enjoy studying. She completed her GSCE's, but as her parents we knew she was cleverer than her results suggested. I thought that once she found a subject she enjoyed she would do better. She decided to go to the boys' grammar school to study A levels but again she had no passion for the subjects she took. Looking back she didn't seem to go to school that much and clearly wanted to grow up and leave school. When she was eighteen she applied to do a children's nursing degree. She didn't appear to have the passion for nursing that I had had but she was good at being with children. She moved away to university digs up in the north of England.

I was very busy at work but missed her enormously. She reported that she enjoyed nursing and was happy. Maybe she had found her forte. We didn't row and I worried about her less and less. Eventually there was a new boyfriend, Ant, whom we gradually got to know, she took and passed her finals and we had a graduation to go to. I found it hard to believe. My baby girl was a fully trained children's nurse. She wanted to be nearer the family and once she had qualified she decided to live with us and work nearer home. She was clearly close to her boyfriend Ant who had decided to train as a teacher. We agreed for them to live together with us and this gave us a year in which to get to know Ant better. Charlotte remained strong and was self-controlled. She had the manner of someone older and I wondered if being the oldest sister had caused her to be like that. It was as if she had been here before. The strong character did have some challenges but I enjoyed them living with us and felt sad when they decided to move out into a flat nearer their work places. I knew it was right for them to move on but I was sad. We had a couple of holidays with them and I tried to introduce them to my favourite pastime, cycling. In the early days they didn't seem interested but now they both love it. Charlotte doesn't race but undertakes lots of sportives (organized cycling events) and is a keen rider.

They decided to get married. As we have three daughters we have always said to them that paying for any wedding is their responsibility. We had paid their living allowance for university, but as marriage arrangements and costs can vary enormously we felt it was best if they decided themselves what they wanted and paid for it themselves. Charlotte and Ant began to plan. They had chosen the venue and began organising the event. It appeared that they wanted it to be everything ours hadn't been. I was a little concerned about the financial considerations but gave myself a talking to. It wasn't my event to make a judgement about the style so I decided not to voice my opinion and to look forward to it. This I did and went to see the venue with them both. I needed a posh outfit to wear and John would need to excel himself as he was father of the bride. The other girls had been asked to be bridesmaids and Josh an usher. It was going to be fun but different from our wedding. Ours cost little and my dress was made by my flatmate. Charlotte planned a flamboyant event much grander than ours.

So my oldest child, my eldest daughter Charlotte was strong and confident. She dealt with difficult situations appropriately and responsibly but you couldn't mess with her. She was settled in her career as a paediatric nurse, was happy with her boyfriend and was going to marry in 2014.

My second child was also a daughter, Hannah. Hannah was different to Charlotte as she was much quieter. However she was also strong but in a different, less dominant way.

She seemed to respond to academic challenges in a more positive manner than Charlotte and appeared to work harder but quietly on her own. She left school with enough qualifications to take a degree. She had always been interested in fundraising. I have a picture of her fundraising at the local children's hospice where I worked at the time. She is sitting in their multisensory room, her eyes alight, keen to make a difference in her fundraising efforts. It was clear that she wanted to move into paid employment in fundraising but wasn't sure how to do it. I remember clearly the day she came home from a university information day. She told me that she had found exactly what she wanted to study for her degree -Event Management. So Hannah set off to study for a degree in Yorkshire. As Charlotte was enjoying Yorkshire and both of us had loved growing up there we thought it a good idea. However Hannah had met a boy, Simon, and clearly living at the other end of the country was not ideal for the relationship. So she moved in her second year to one of the London Universities and managed to obtain her degree.

It wasn't as easy for Hannah to get into work after qualifying. She applied to lots of charities for fundraising posts. Each time she went for interview she was told she had lost out to someone with experience. It was very exciting when Hannah went for an interview at a hospice in London. However I was concerned that she still hadn't got experience. I suggested that if she wasn't successful she should offer to volunteer, to be helpful but also gain valuable experience. It happened again but this time she managed to obtain a volunteering role. After a few months Hannah was able to apply for a post and successfully gain paid employment.

Hannah is much prettier than I have ever been. She is the sort of person who could wear a bin liner and look great. She has high standards and learns a lot by looking at others. She decides what is good and bad about any situation. I often realise she is just observing others, seeing how they react and using the information appropriate for any future events. Hannah is still seeing Simon, her first real boyfriend. However their relationship is different from mine with John. If Hannah or Simon wants to do something they just do it even if the other doesn't want to. For example Hannah wanted to go to Florida with the family. Simon didn't feel it was what he wanted to do and Hannah went anyway. It's the same the other way round, too.

Hannah is adventurous and takes some well-controlled risks. For example she carries out some daring leisure activities; she has done parachuting and skydiving. She has undertaken some long distance cycle rides such as London to Amsterdam. When she has an event planned she borrows my trainer and plans her training schedule. I get the feeling that she carries this out and is successful because of it. She cycles to work most days and this keeps her fit and saves enormous amounts of money. I asked John, this morning, how Hannah should be described and he said 'adventurous'. She is certainly that. When she was at school she applied for World Challenge as her sister Charlotte had. World Challenge involves children going to far reaching parts of the world but taking responsibility themselves for fundraising for some of the costs. Some community work is included in the trip as well as climbing and walking across the continent. Hannah went to Brazil and undertook some support work planting trees in the rain forests. I have never done such an exciting thing and it gave me the idea to enter long distance cycle events. I also wanted to do some of the things they had done.

Hannah is also very accommodating. I notice that she doesn't judge people unnecessarily. She is good with our ex-foster son and some of her friends have special needs of varying sorts.

Joshua is a challenging character to write about, mainly because he presents himself in one way but is actually not really like this. He is very, very funny with a dry sense of humour.

Josh has had a few challenges in life. I remember taking him to visit his primary school before he started aged four. The teacher was asking what he was interested in. Over recent weeks he had been looking at drain-pipes on the houses we walked past. He was tracing where the water flowed and several times we needed to stop and look together, tracing where the water would go. I told the teacher this because I found it fascinating that a child of four was interested in such things. There was suddenly a scream from Josh. While exploring the class area he had come across the toilet block and noticed the cistern was not just above the pan as it was at home. It was raised and sat high above it on the wall. He was intrigued by this and spent a while working it out, much to the interest of the teacher.

Josh didn't really settle at school. It became more and more noticeable that he was struggling. Parents' evening led us to believe that he was behind other children of his age. Yet at home we felt his interests and interactions were actually normal if not slightly advanced. In the end the school wanted him to have extra support and he was assessed. It was decided that he needed a statement to the effect that he would benefit from one to one support in school. He had some lovely workers assigned to him who helped him over the years.

Josh loved swimming and was well ahead of the children in his class who were taking their 10 metre badge. He was up to his 1000 metre badge and caused havoc in school because the class couldn't wait for him to swim it, so a lovely teaching assistant volunteered to stay with him and walk him back to school.

Josh is also kind and I remember that at a school second-hand sale shortly after Sarah was born the teachers said that Josh was the only child in the school who had spent his money on someone else. He had bought his baby sister a book. A later example of his thoughtfulness concerns his grandfather. When my father was a child he had read that a total eclipse of the sun was due to occur when he was a mature adult. He waited all his life to see it. When the time arrived we all travelled to Northern France to get a reasonable view.

Imagine my father's disappointment when the day clouded over and we didn't see the sun, let alone an eclipse. Josh reassured my dad "Don't worry, Grandad, when I am a man I will take you to see an eclipse." I don't think my father thought it would happen. However just before my accident there was a total eclipse in Australia. As promised Josh offered to go with my dad aged 79.They had 3 weeks away together. I can't actually remember their return home but understand that it was a fantastic time away and a memory Josh will have forever.

Josh hated any school work that involved writing and we knew his special needs would affect him as he grew. We had heard that a secondary school was available for dyslexic children in Broadstairs, Kent. We tried to get him a place there but lost the tribunal case and instead he was sent to a large state school. Despite our serious concerns the teachers there understood Josh and his special needs and the school proved to be perfect for him. However he was a shy boy and when he applied to Tesco for a part time job and gained an interview I was worried that he might not cope. Yet he got the job and has continued there ever since he was 16. He worked as an email shopper but when a special venue for this was created in another area Josh couldn't travel there, so he stayed at the one near our home and changed to stacking shelves and eventually working on the till.

Despite not doing that well in his GCSE's Josh always worked hard and began to develop further in the sixth form, so that he achieved reasonable results in the end, winning a place at college to study computing. We were delighted with his progress and thrilled that he felt able to apply for a degree. He didn't move away but studied at the local university, continuing to work at Tesco. He was about to hand in his dissertation when my accident happened.

In some ways Sarah was different from the others but I guess her upbringing was different. In many respects it felt as if she had five parents, each playing a part in her upbringing and making a significant difference to it. She was a lovely baby and we all enjoyed her presence greatly. I could see she had a little bit of each of them within her.

She was also a good swimmer and we spent a lot of time travelling to and from the swimming pool. Sarah announced when she was five that she thought she was grammar school material. It surprised me that she didn't actually win a place but the others had done so well without going that I wasn't concerned. We felt that she would be successful as she is intellectually very able. I do wonder what she will choose to do in life. She is able enough to choose to be whatever she wants. She became a bit interested in cycling when she was fifteen - we bought her a time trial bike and she entered a few races.

She is also kind and I have seen her supporting others but she hates dealing with anything medical and knows this would prevent her from being a doctor. She says "I hate blood". It is impossible to discuss anything medical in her presence as she just screams. So she is very different to her sister Charlotte who is now nursing. However Sarah can sort out other problems and uses logic to help her plan solutions appropriately. Like Hannah and Josh, Sarah likes adventures and she is already undertaking challenge events like climbing Ben Nevis. She has good friends who she spends time with and who gave her much support when I was less stable.

So we feel very lucky to have four children of our own and J G who is still part of our family. They all have their own lives but you get the feeling that they care about each other greatly. We tend to spend time at our home all together, like at Christmas when Charlotte and Ant will stay and often Hannah and Simon will be with us for some of the day. We play family games together and usually enjoy each other's company. We went away a lot cycling and the children coped with it.

Obviously the children are massively important to me and have remained vital during my long recovery.

John has been my partner for many years. In fact he has been my only significant partner. We have both changed dramatically over our time together and our relationship has changed. However we have coped with these changes well and are still together. I am not aware of any episodes that have significantly challenged the relationship. There are harder days that all people go through, but on the whole we have sorted things out and moved forward together.

When I broke my leg on the trampoline John wasn't very good to me. He seemed unaware of how difficult it all was and would happily watch me hop all over the house in my efforts to keep the children cared for and the house clean and tidy. He didn't ever help me and I am awkward and refused to ask him for help. The result was I was angry at his inability to see what a struggle everything was and therefore his lack of support and care wasn't good.

However I wasn't good to him when years later he broke his leg skiing. I wonder if I was still angry with him for his lack of support years before. When he was on the mountain with a broken ankle I was horrible to him. He seemed to make a meal of it and didn't do anything in the house while his leg was in plaster for six weeks. We did not seem able to help each other if the other was unwell or hurt - not an ideal situation for a married couple to be in. However when I had my major accident John was clearly fantastic to me over a long period of time and I am a lucky woman to have someone who has supported me so well.

So my marriage was good and we were enjoying a bit more time together as the children were growing and building their own lives.

My parents remained important to me. They lived close by and we saw them regularly but they weren't dependent on me or me on them. They had busy and fulfilling lives and regularly went abroad for extended periods of time. They had a house in southern France as well as one locally. We spent many holidays in their French home. We loved to take our cycles and explore. Sometimes we met them in France and sometimes we went alone. We were aware that as they grew older it would become harder to see them regularly and maybe hard work and commitment would be needed in the future. Clearly we loved them and would do what was necessary or required by them. Of course I never thought that it would end up being the other way round and it would be me that needed extensive care. However at the time they were in fine health, and indeed still are. We enjoyed their company but in reality we all had busy lives and before the accident didn't see that much of each other.

I also have a brother Alan. We have never fallen out but over time have followed our own paths in life and have gone years without seeing each other at all. Alan has also lived in France but has recently returned and lives and works in England as a countryside warden.

John has a natural sister and two adopted siblings. We see them all but spend more time with Sarah, his little sister, and their two young children Kyan and Asher.

CHAPTER SIX
HOW AND WHY I CAME TO WRITE THIS

So now you know all about me prior to the accident. I have told you a little about my family. Next I am going to tell you about what happened to us. I believe that it's right to say 'us' as the experience was challenging for us all and I want to acknowledge how difficult it has been for all my family. In fact in many ways it's been a harder time for them than it has for me. Clearly I have absolutely no memory for about four months around the incident so it's difficult for me to write about it. In my mind all that happened could be the imagination of my family. I don't remember anything. When I began to come round I was aware that I was in hospital and that I had been there a long time. That is my first memory.

So in order to write this I have spoken to each of my children and they're going to tell you their story.

Obviously each of my children had similar experiences dealing with what happened to me. However they are unique individuals with their own thoughts and experiences. I don't want to be repetitive when I relay what happened to each of them. Equally I want to give them each the opportunity to express how it was for them as individuals.

When I got to the stage of exploring what happened to each of them, I started writing what Hannah told me. We found that my communication, note taking and memory skills were now limited. So we developed a system whereby she would give me small instalments by phone as she travelled to work. I would then write it down using a speech to text software program called Dragon. Once it was documented, I sent it to Hannah who played with it and then sent it back to me.

I had wanted to write down my experiences for some time. I felt it was going to be therapeutic for me as I slowly came to terms with what had happened. I also thought it would be good for my children to have a record and maybe it would be helpful to others in a similar situation.

I knew that to make it readable I would need some major help as I have some problems with punctuation and grammar now. I had asked various people to help but they had thought it was not a good idea for me to undertake such a task and therefore were not keen to be involved. I was explaining this to Karen, someone I used to work with a few years ago. I genuinely wasn't telling her because I was asking for her help as I had all but given up on the idea at that stage. However Karen offered to help! She has been fantastic. I regularly email her a section, she works with it and then emails it back when she has tidied it up. I couldn't have embarked on this without her support. I wish to thank her sincerely. It's also an example of how I have found, since the accident, that you don't always realise who is important to you. Some of the friends I had considered very special before the accident haven't actually been that great since. However there are others, like Karen, who I clearly liked but saw less regularly, who have been a major support for me when I needed it. The point I am making is that you don't necessarily know who's vital to you.

Once Hannah's experience was written down I realised she had described events which were obviously very similar to the experiences of the other three siblings. She has given a fairly comprehensive account, so for the other three I have focused on their individual thoughts and views, rather than facts and events. I have also included (in the appendix) a copy of the diary that Charlotte encouraged them to write as it shows what they were all thinking at the actual time. You will notice that the girls appear keen to write and write a lot. However with severe dyslexia Josh doesn't like writing and in many ways is less keen to express himself verbally. So his input is limited compared with his sisters. Yet in his own way he has been so supportive to me- he has encouraged me to drive forward by ignoring what I can't do and only focusing on what I can do, if I try hard enough. He has continued to show his lovely dry sense of humour, for example focusing on asking me to do a back flip when I was ventilated and unconscious. It's significant that the first documentation of me joining in and interacting normally with the family was when I smiled at his joke about the back flip.

Each child of mine has made a unique and special contribution to my recovery. They all have different strengths but I know I would have struggled to cope without them. What a lucky woman I am.

People moan about young people today. Not me!

Without them and all their friends it would have been so much more difficult for me to come to terms with what has happened.

I have now written each of their stories for you to read.

CHAPTER SEVEN – THE CHILDREN'S CONTRIBUTIONS

Hannah

Whilst out with her housemates Hannah received an odd text message from her father saying 'Any news?' She hadn't been expecting any news so she didn't think much of it and when she didn't get a response to 'What do you mean?' she thought that maybe her dad had sent it to the wrong person and she quickly forgot about it. A few days later she was at work -she uses a mobile phone for work activities but wouldn't normally answer a personal call in work time. However this call was from her father and she knew we were in Tenerife on a cycling holiday. She answered. Her dad asked her if she was with friends and she thought that he wanted a private conversation without anyone being able to listen. She told him she was with other people but could move away to have a private conversation and he answered 'No that's OK. You are better with others.' He then started crying and she realised something serious was happening. At first she couldn't make much sense of him. She knew her younger sister Sarah was skiing and felt she must have been injured. However after a few moments Hannah was able to make out that her mum had had a serious accident cycling. Judging by her dad's emotion she was expecting the worst. When she enquired her dad replied, 'It doesn't look good.' In the next few moments she was to learn that her mum had been in a coma for three days already. Her dad told her that as Sarah was skiing with the school she mustn't tell anyone at all in case someone put it on Facebook and Sarah found out. He really wanted Sarah to be told in a sensitive way. Clearly

Hannah was distressed but fortunately her work colleagues were very supportive. They offered to drive her back to Kent. She agreed but wasn't sure what to do next. She felt that this sort of thing sometimes happened to other people but not to you. It felt unreal. Her colleague and friend tried to comfort her by saying, 'I'm sure she'll be fine.' Hannah replied, 'I work at a hospice- I know what can happen.'

By this time Charlotte had also been told by John and spoke to Hannah by phone. They agreed to meet up at the family home in Maidstone. Hannah, or her work colleague, thought that getting her passport was a sensible idea. So a senior colleague drove her home to get it and then on to Maidstone, a good hour's drive away.

Once home Charlotte and Hannah supported each other and discussed what to do next. Josh was also at home. It was agreed that they wanted to fly to Tenerife. John had hinted that this was a poor idea because it left Sarah unsupported when she came home. So they decided that two of them would go the next day and one would stay behind to tell Sarah when she got off the school coach several days later. Hannah didn't really want to stay as she wanted to see her mum and be with her dad. He clearly needed support. Of course none of them wanted to stay behind but they all recognised it was important that one of them did.

There was a discussion about who would be best to tell Sarah. Hannah said that she thought Sarah would like Charlotte to do it as she was calm and sensible but would also be compassionate. Somehow she had the ability to show she was very distressed but at the same time to remain sensible. Also, her nursing experience had given her practice in having difficult conversations with people. They all agreed this was right and Charlotte volunteered to stay in England and travel out later with Sarah.

Hannah has said that Charlotte had come home without her passport. She would obviously need this so together the three of them decided to drive to Charlotte's home and get it. So off they went, all together, not really understanding what they were all facing but feeling it important to collect the passport in order to be doing something. They drove in one car to Charlotte's house. On the way back to Maidstone, they realised that they had not eaten. It was very late so they stopped at a McDonalds which they were driving past and had a meal. Hannah has said that this became a common experience. They spent time eating food simply to feel full - it wasn't important to Hannah where or what she ate. McDonalds was easy and they often went to one in Tenerife. She says for many days in a row this was her typical diet.

Charlotte's boyfriend, Ant, worked hard at getting the travel arrangements to Tenerife organised. The cheapest way for them all to get there was to buy a package holiday- Ant duly found one but it necessitated travelling from Leeds. Arrangements were made for Hannah and Josh to go and stay with John's sister Sarah as she lives near Leeds in Bradford. Hannah said that Josh was very sensible and calm. He honestly thought it would all be all right in the end. His calm optimism helped Hannah cope.

Hannah said that eventually she got to sleep and the next day travelled to Bradford with Josh. They were helped enormously by Sarah and her husband Roger who drove them to the airport. Sarah's children were also helpful because they expressed sadness about what was happening but were also getting on with their lives.

Hannah had a little incident as she mislaid her luggage at the airport, and only realised it was missing just prior to boarding. Luckily the airport staff gave her help and support in finding it. While Hannah and Josh were at the airport waiting for their flight Hannah remembers a lady asking them if they were going somewhere nice on holiday. Hannah told me it was a particularly difficult question to answer. They didn't want to embarrass the lady and it wasn't her fault for asking but equally it was very difficult to answer in any way other than embarrass her and tell the truth. Hannah thinks she managed without saying the first time she was asked but subsequently did tell people who asked. It was just easier than not telling them. Hannah told me that was the first time she had ever flown when she wasn't going on holiday somewhere nice and exciting and it was clearly a big difference. When she got to Tenerife they were met by her dad and the cycle coach who had very kindly taken time away from coaching to support them. She helped Hannah and Josh check into the hotel. Fortunately there was Wi-Fi and Hannah said how important that was as there were lots of emails and Facebook friends constantly asking how I was and whether there any sign of improvement. At that time there was no sign at all.

John had a significant problem accessing any money. Although Hannah was unable to help with that problem she could offer other practical help. The first evening Hannah and Josh were there they decided to go for a walk. They really did not know what to do with themselves so they walked and walked. Eventually they decided to get some food and found a Chinese restaurant. It was nice but in Hannah's mind it was going to cost a lot if they ate out regularly. So they went to a corner shop to buy provisions. They bought some plastic cups to drink from but also put cereal in them. Hannah has a nice photo of John eating his breakfast. Hannah told me that in the shop they were again asked if they were on holiday. Hannah shook her head hoping that would be the end of it but the shop owner pressed on. 'Oh, are you here on business?' he said. Once again Hannah shook her head, knowing now that that was not going to be the end of it. After an awkward silence, John explained that I was in intensive care and that I was in a coma. Coincidentally the shop manager told them that he knew the intensive care unit I was in as a family member had been cared for very recently and had survived. He told them they had survived because he had prayed. He told John, Hannah and Josh that they should also pray for me. He knew that if they did it 11 or 24 times a day I would be OK! He quickly jotted down the prayer (at this point a queue had started forming at the till) and insisted that John recited every word out loud. Hannah told me that although she doesn't have any faith she found this particularly interesting. Partly because seeing her dad pray to Hindu gods seemed such a strange concept to her and partly because she thought 'I will do anything to get my mum back', she decided to google the prayer and learn it. It was something the whole family chanted to each other over the coming weeks. It also meant a lot that a stranger cared for our family enough to add his own particular support. When the man got John to say the prayer out loud Hannah was amused by the thought of what I would say if I could see John praying. Hannah also made sure that the prayer was downloaded onto her iPhone so she could play it to me.

Om Sai Ram

Om Sai namoh namah
Shri Sai namoh namah
Jai Jai Sai namoh namah
Satguru Sai namoh namah

The days were long for them all because they were only allowed to visit at lunchtime and at 6 pm. If they went at lunchtime they didn't have anywhere to go before the evening session. So they ended up just visiting in the evening and hanging about in the day.

Hannah and Josh made their way to the hospital on the first day. John told them that they would be allowed into the room at 7pm but as they did not want to miss any visiting time they left with lots of time to spare and arrived one hour early.

They agreed that they should go straight up and sign in before finding somewhere to get a drink. Hannah explained that it was so lucky they did that because John had got the time wrong and if they had turned up at 7pm they would have missed the visiting hour as it was actually at 6 o'clock. (It was very unusual for John to get the timing wrong. Hannah explained that she thought he must have been relying on the cycle coach a lot of the time before they arrived.)

Hannah told how John stopped them outside the room and explained what to expect when they went in. John told them that I had had my head shaved and that I was very swollen all over. My face had been destroyed but the surgeons had done a very good job at sewing me up. He also explained that there were tubes in my nose and mouth and lots of machines. Hannah went in first with John and remembers being thankful that John had prepared her. As it was she was not shocked but was actually relieved. She said I looked younger and surprisingly healthy. Then she explained how I started to move. Although I was still ventilated and unconscious I was not lying still. I was thrashing about and restless. Hannah looked at John immediately and wondered why he had not mentioned the thrashing, but when she saw John's face she immediately knew this was new! John took this as a very good sign and tried to get some answers from the doctors but didn't get much. They just agreed that I was moving a lot. Hannah wasn't sure if it was a good sign. She looked on the internet for information about restlessness in unconscious patients but none of the information she read actually said what, if anything, it meant. All people seemed to respond differently but it made her realise how serious it was likely to be. For example she read about Ozzy Osbourne who had been unconscious for 12 hours. It seemed that your brain would be affected by loss of consciousness in the long term and you were unlikely to be the same person ever again. The next day they visited and I was still again.

There was quite a problem getting accurate medical information when you were distressed and didn't speak any Spanish. The doctors and nurses were obviously looking after me well but they couldn't communicate information to my family who must have been so unsure about what was happening.

A few days later Sarah and Charlotte flew into Tenerife and Hannah, Josh and John met them at the airport. Hannah said that she knew the plane had arrived and could see the girls through the glass wall but they didn't seem to be collecting their luggage like the other passengers. Hannah couldn't understand what they were playing at. Couldn't they hurry? It seemed to take a ridiculously long time. However when they came through into the arrivals hall Hannah realised what the problem was. Their luggage had been lost by the airline. They had nothing!

It seems fairly stressful to find yourself abroad with no belongings. However it was a problem that almost faded into insignificance alongside what else they were facing.

They checked in at their hotel which turned out to be very basic- Hannah said the mirror was lined with tiny spiders. The staff there didn't seem particularly helpful but eventually gave them a new 'spider free' room. The hotel also had no Wi-Fi which Hannah felt was essential at this time as so many people were trying to get in touch. Subsequently many hours were spent in Hannah, Josh and John's hotel with the five of them trying to squeeze onto three beds.

John explained to Charlotte and Sarah that they had missed visiting hours that day (visiting hours in intensive care were extremely strict, the doors were locked and there was no one to speak to), so they decided to go and get some dinner. McDonald's was opposite the hotel and easy and cheap. As they had all spent money on the flights and hotel, and Charlotte and her fiancé had even had to find the money for Sarah's flight, they resolved that they were all happy to go somewhere cheap and easy. It was at McDonalds that John told Sarah and Charlotte what had happened. John explained how he had finished the day's cycle and was waiting for the keys from the second group (that I was in). He told them about the phone call that he had received from the cycle group explaining that I was in trouble. He said that he cycled back and could see two ambulances, but when he tried to see me he was waved away (this was apparently one hour after the initial phone call). He went back to the room and gathered some clothes for me, expecting to pick me up and take me home. He made his way to the hospital where no-one spoke English and no-one warned him before he walked into a room and saw someone who couldn't exactly be identified as his wife. He eventually realised that it was me - my head had been shaved and my face was almost completely unrecognizable. He then spent the next three days trying to find out if there was any news to ring the children and tell them what was going on but there was no improvement. Clearly it was distressing for them all but Sarah became particularly distressed and couldn't eat any of her food.

Before Charlotte and Sarah flew out Charlotte had had the idea of buying a blank book to be written in by the family as they were by my bedside. She had had experience of such a diary being kept when a patient was unconscious and felt that this might be a good idea. So it was started and has remained very important to me.

Hannah told Charlotte that I was restless even though unconscious. They discussed whether this was good or not.The next day when they visited I was very still again.

Hannah remembers having an in depth conversation about what they would do if I was to die. They were sunbathing on the garden roof area of the hotel, high above the streets. The conversation focused on how great it would be if I could survive. Neither of them dared to imagine that I would return to the Mum they used to have. But if I could at least survive, how fantastic would that be. They discussed how they would feel if I ended up very disabled. Hannah told me that Charlotte had commented that she hoped I would at least be well enough to wipe my own bum. They both laughed. Charlotte reassured Hannah that she would give up working as a nurse to care for me instead.

The next day they decided not to spend the whole day waiting for visiting hours at the hospital. They had been spending the whole time waiting in one of the hotel rooms but decided that was probably not what I would have wanted. Hannah had been to Tenerife the previous year on holiday and knew that there was a very good water park on the island, but she said although she had suggested it to the others it didn't feel like a good idea. She couldn't imagine enjoying the attractions as she had the previous year. After a quick Google search they found there was a museum so they spent the morning there. They all enjoyed going out together and Hannah remembers seeing a mummy in the museum. She read that the average life span at that time was 35 years – by that measure I had actually had a long, fulfilling life. She was trying to see the positives as much as possible.

After their day out they resumed their normal positions on the three beds in the hotel room where they all connected to Wi-Fi and continued to respond to worried friends and family asking questions. Hannah had been warned not to search for information on line but she found some comfort in scouring the internet looking for positive stories. She could not find much and what little there was seemed extremely vague, but she did read advice to 'stay positive' around someone unconscious as that might give them the mental strength to keep fighting for their life. Charlotte had told Hannah that she didn't feel it was acceptable to cry or be distressed in my hearing. So the four of them made a pact that they would not cry but would leave the room if they felt they were going to.

Hannah also read stories of people waking up after listening to their favourite music tracks. She had read that hearing was thought to be the last sense to disappear when a patient is unconscious, so they decided to download some music onto their phones and play it to me when they visited. These included James Blunt 'Three wise men', Katie Melua 'Ninety nine red balloons' and Les Mis 'I dreamed a dream' among others. Hannah recalls Charlotte putting the earpiece in my ear. Apparently I looked as if I heard and I started to move my left hand ever so slightly, so Charlotte started to sing with the recording. It made Charlotte cry and as agreed she left the room so if I could hear I wouldn't be distressed. They all kept that pact while I was so unwell, although it was hard at times. When she returned to the hospital bed, she played a song from Les Mis but apparently I didn't respond to this at all so they quickly changed the track back to Katie Melua and I started moving my hand again.

Hannah also talks about the language barrier being a significant problem. They didn't really know how bad I was as the doctors could not speak English very well and they weren't really getting any updates. I think they made assumptions and guessed a little. It was infrequently that they actually spoke to someone. The background I come from is palliative care, care of the dying. In Britain family members are seen as part of the team (if the patient wants this). They are kept fully informed of what is going on and can visit when it is best for the patient. It appears it was very different in Tenerife's intensive care. My family felt they had to keep to the strict visiting hours, so they left late afternoon and didn't know how I was until they arrived in the afternoon the following day. It was hard to arrange to see a doctor and wasn't always really helpful anyway. Once the doctor could only say "poor" and "not good" and they didn't know what that meant! A poor day or my long-term future was poor? They made much use of Google to get information about head injury but learnt that it varies so much from person to person. Some people do well but others don't and you can't always tell who going to do well and who isn't. It seemed you couldn't tell at this stage.

Hannah thought about the future. In the short term I had booked loads of activities. One event was my father's 80th birthday. I had booked a house for us all to share in Southwold to celebrate his birthday. It was very expensive but I felt we should celebrate such an important occasion in style. We were also cycling to Amsterdam with Hannah and her boyfriend Simon. We had booked the ferry and the hotels. I had also booked a London theatre trip for us all. They all needed cancelling. The biggest problem was that we had booked and paid for a trip to Florida. As there are four offspring who are now adults with commitments, I had found it was becoming less likely that we could all go on holiday together. So we had booked a trip for all of us for three weeks in the summer of 2013. This was an attempt at all being together for a holiday, potentially for the last time. We had all been saving and had paid for the flights and lodgings. John had just bought the Disney tickets which made us all feel we were getting closer to going. For two years we had so looked forward to this trip and now it seemed unlikely it would happen. We had actually booked two years earlier because we needed time to save. Should we go if our mum has died? Hannah was thinking about this. She knew I would want them to go and enjoy the holiday but Hannah knew it would be spoilt.

Hannah also worried about work and being able to be with me. The intensive care had said that they needed some-one in Tenerife at all times. She felt that if I was ventilated for a long time I would need someone with me in case I came round. What would it be like for me if there was no-one to speak to me if I suddenly gained consciousness? She decided that she would come to see me in Tenerife at Easter, her next booked annual leave. In her mind she was trying to make sure I wouldn't be left alone. She knew my parents were also coming over and she felt they all needed to get together and sort out a plan to prevent me being alone.

She felt she must stop feeling sorry for herself. She wrote that in the diary. She felt lucky to be in a position where there was a chance I might live. Other people had to cope when death had occurred. How lucky to be in a position where it might not happen. She tried to think what I would want if I could say anything. She knew that I would want them to be able to cope and get on with a fun life. She felt at this point that she had enjoyed her childhood. She felt that we had a good relationship and that wouldn't change even if I died. She felt lucky to have had me as a mum and she had no regrets about our relationship. All these thoughts would always stay with her whatever happened. This helped her, at the time, as it gave her positive things to think about. Of course I don't remember that she was thinking these amazing things but as I hear her now and write her thoughts down I feel so proud of her and indeed of them all in different ways! I feel especially proud of them for the pact they made because it must have been very hard for them to carry it out and if by any chance I had any awareness it would have made a huge difference to me.

Hannah received an email encouraging her to apply for a new job but she thought what my advice would be. "Stay in the job you have got for a while. You still have loads to learn." Even though she couldn't ask me she felt my advice was present. She had been told that John had agreed that I was given a tracheotomy. She felt that it might be a bad sign. Did it mean that I wouldn't get better? However when she saw me after I had been to theatre she thought it looked a lot better and strangely more comfortable for me. I didn't have too many tubes coming out of my mouth and nose and my breathing seemed easier. Having worried beforehand she was actually pleased for me, once she saw it, and thought it was best for me that it had been done. Hannah felt that it was probably bad news really because they had asked a doctor whether my coma was drug induced. He had said no, that they had tried me without drugs for a few days and there was no sign of response from me. I think they had hoped that my coma was induced by drugs in order to allow my brain to heal. When they heard this wasn't the case they were more concerned.

Sarah

As you're aware, Sarah was on a skiing holiday with school when it happened. She had had a fantastic holiday and one that she would always remember. She was returning to school in the coach, tired from the journey but very happy with her friends. She saw a car in the school car park that was our small car and she wandered over to it. She wasn't particularly surprised to see Charlotte as the driver and she put her bag in the back. After asking if Sarah had had a good holiday, Charlotte went on to tell her that she had some very bad news. Sarah thought it was going to be about J G. She noticed that Charlotte was crying and distressed. Sarah remembers asking 'What is it?' and Charlotte told her that I had had a cycling accident. Sarah asked her how bad and was told, 'Very bad. She is in a coma.' Sarah asked if I would live and Charlotte said 'We don't know.'

Sarah said they were both silent. They drove home. When they got home Charlotte said they were going to go to Tenerife the next day. 'We are going to be near Mum.' Charlotte told Sarah to pack a bag as they were leaving immediately. Sarah told me that she can't really remember much about that evening but she remembers she rang a friend to tell her and found this useful. Charlotte's house, which is an hour's drive away, was where they planned to stay before the flight the next day. When they arrived they ordered some take-away food. The girls wanted to sleep together and so Charlotte's boyfriend got sent to sleep on the sofa. Sarah said that she fell asleep quickly. She doesn't have any memory of getting to the airport or how she coped with the situation. She does remember sitting and crying on the plane. She also remembers the lost luggage challenge. She so wanted to see her Dad, Hannah and Josh and the luggage problem was just causing delay. She was glad when it was over and wasn't concerned she now had no clothes to wear. She was just pleased to be with her family.

Like Hannah, Sarah found the hotel dirty and lacking Wi-Fi. She said they had an ongoing joke about the standard of the hotels, each of them claiming theirs was actually the best. Although Sarah's hotel had no Wi-Fi it did serve a good breakfast and she remembers them taking a photo, on their phone, of breakfast and sending it to the others to show off.

Sarah found the conversation with John at McDonalds very difficult. She was told my face was badly damaged and I looked very unpleasant. Sarah doesn't like blood and she didn't feel that she was going to be able to face seeing me so disfigured. It triggered her distress and she couldn't eat any of the food.

The next day Sarah visited the hospital to see for herself what I was like. She felt my face was bad but it was strangely OK compared to what she had feared. My hair had been shaved off and Sarah thought it looked all right. (She was used to my long hair which I often tied back. Now I had none.) Sarah has struggled to remember much of what happened in Tenerife as she appears to have blocked a lot of it out. However she does remember feeling how helpful her brother and sisters were. They were all coping with a major challenge together and she found that comforting. She remembers a lot of hanging around waiting to see me. When she did see me she felt rushed as the others were waiting their turn. She felt that I would live, although she knows she didn't have any facts to base this feeling on but just felt it inside. She knew I would probably end up handicapped but didn't know and couldn't imagine what this actually would mean to me or to her. Her main memory was visiting with John, the day after the tracheotomy. He went to speak to the doctor and Sarah went into my room alone. I was propped up and staring at her strangely. Something had changed. I wasn't being ventilated. She said she was so very scared. "I ran out crying and screaming. I realised I scared the others and they assumed you had died." Sarah told Charlotte, who reassured her that it looked like a good sign. Sarah said, "We went back in to see you and realised Charlotte was right but you were looking, yet didn't seem to be seeing anything, although you were staring." She obviously found this unsettling.

Sarah told me, "I knew the others wanted to stay in Tenerife with you but to be honest I wanted to get back to home life. It was important for me to be at school as this was a normal thing to do."

Sarah was due to take her mock GCSE exams shortly and she knew I would encourage her still to take them so she wanted to do well. So Sarah was very happy to return home and hoped I would get back to England in the future or she would return to see me soon.

Charlotte

These are Charlotte's own words.

"OK, so where to begin? I don't think as an adult I have ever written something I wasn't forced to write (nursing notes etc.)!

I was merrily eating dinner in the local Harvester restaurant when I received an odd text from my mum's phone asking if I had got home to Josh yet as there was something I needed to be told. I jokingly sent a text back 'Has Dad broken his arm again?' as in recent trips my parents had made, my dad always managed to feign some kind of pathetic injury. The answer was of course 'No, when will you get home?' to which I jokingly replied 'Is Mum pregnant?'

I subsequently wonder what Dad was thinking at receiving this text, knowing that my mum was in a critical condition in ITU. Again, the answer skirted around the edge of finding out if everyone was OK and urging me to go home and be with my brother.

At this point I realised there was something wrong, so we paid for our meal and rushed back to my parents' house where we were asked to call my dad. Josh promptly came out of his bedroom and phoned Dad on speaker phone. This is when we were told of my mother's accident and subsequent condition in hospital.

I don't particularly recall the exact words used in the conversation between the three of us. However, I do remember Josh saying 'Is it bad?' and my dad becoming audibly choked and just saying 'Yes'.

The next little bit is a whirlwind but in summary Hannah came home from work as she had been told the news there and we went about making rushed plans with budget airlines to get us all out to Tenerife to be with my mother, but also to support my dad in what must have been horrific for him.

Obviously the first hurdle to tackle was to work out how and when Sarah was to be told. At this point she was somewhere in Italy skiing with the school and was not due back until Saturday (it's currently Wednesday). All manner of options were considered, including driving to the ski resort in Italy and bringing her home from there or even flying to Tenerife from there.

Dad was insistent she was not to be told by a teacher and have to endure the end of the trip and a 20 hour coach trip home with that knowledge. We had offers from Grandad and a close family friend, Sheila, to pick Sarah up and tell her but both Josh and I really thought one of us should be there for her and break the news.

Hannah was very keen to go to Tenerife straight away and so it was left for me and Josh to decide who should stay to break the news to Sarah. In the end we came to the conclusion that it would be best if I were the one to do this- I felt that she would find it easier to embrace me if that was what she needed. I also felt that I had my husband-to-be at home to support me whereas Josh would be on his own while he waited for Sarah's return.

So my brother and sister set off to Tenerife while I waited for Sarah to get back to break the news. News from my dad was very limited. He was obviously in shock and found it hard to talk over the phone so my mother's condition was pretty unknown. It became a lot clearer to me how she was once Hannah and Josh had arrived as Hannah described in detail what Mum looked like, how she moved and behaved etc. I feel that my siblings' arrival in Tenerife greatly benefited my dad as he then had some support and was more able to talk about my mum.

The day came when Sarah was due to arrive home from her school trip. I had wanted to go alone to tell her. She got off the school bus, I greeted her and we hauled the most awkward shaped, huge, massively over-packed and heavy bag into my Ka. She then sat in the front passenger seat next to me. This is when I told her 'Mum has had an accident, she is in a coma in Tenerife.... We are booked on a flight first thing tomorrow to go and see her.' Sarah looked shocked and said 'How bad is it?' and I replied 'Bad'. She leant over and hugged me and cried on the way home.

From here it was a bit of a rush to get her packed and to drive to my house in Leatherhead as this was nearer to Gatwick airport for our flight next morning. That night we feasted on pizza and chicken.

At the airport I decided to buy Sarah a set of pens and a beautiful writing book of her choice. With my background as a nurse it was often something we filled in for children who had been very ill in intensive care so that they (hopefully) could read it later. Writing in such a book also helped the families to feel they were doing something for their relative.

Arriving in Tenerife was at least warm. It was good to see my family but we were too late for visiting hours that day so we checked into our rank, spider-infested room (which Hannah managed to get changed for us with some amazing Spanglish) and headed for McDonalds. This was to become our second home due to its free and reliable Wi-Fi!

Seeing Mum for the first time was a shock. As we were only allowed in two at a time we developed an order of arrival with two people starting (me and Hannah) and then Sarah replacing Hannah. I don't know why but it seemed important to Sarah that when she first saw Mum she was with me. This made sense to me as with my nursing background I felt I was best placed to answer her questions should she have any. However I also felt that I wanted to see Mum before supporting Sarah as I didn't want my reaction to affect hers and wanted time to understand what was going on.

I was shocked when I saw Mum. Although Hannah had described it in great detail nothing can really prepare you. Mum was completely bald and swollen all over which made her look so young and beautiful because her skin was tight and pearlescent. On her left side there were no visible injuries but as you walked round to the other side of the room you could see the injury she sustained to her lip was quite extensive.

The care my mum received in Tenerife was, in my opinion, amazing. She was always immaculate with crisp sheets. Sadly I feel that she actually got better care abroad than she would have done in the UK. Although I was happy and confident that the hospital was doing their best to help my mum, the language barrier was a problem. None of the nurses could speak any English and there was just one German doctor who had mastered basic English. I was frustrated that there was not a translator as there was in the hospitals in 'Sun, Sea and A&E'.

With my nursing knowledge and a bit of nosiness I managed to ascertain that Mum wasn't being sedated. She had paracetamol running through a long line and an NG tube with what looked like 'chocolate milk' going through. Dad joked that she would hate to be force fed chocolate milk as she always had a problem with her weight and was meticulous about her diet, particularly now she was cycling so much. With my understanding I felt this wasn't good news. I had been under the impression that she was in an induced coma to prevent extensive brain injury due to swelling etc, but with the knowledge that her coma was not induced I began to lose hope.

Hannah spent hours trawling the internet reading miracle stories of people who suddenly woke up from uninduced comas and were fine. I, however, having told many a family not to do what Hannah was currently doing, tried to remain what I like to call 'realistic'.

One morning the German doctor explained (as best he could) that Mum really wasn't making the progress they had hoped for. He asked if we would consent to Mum having a tracheostomy tube inserted to make her more comfortable. This, I explained to my family, would leave Mum's mouth free and would be much more comfortable for her. So it was agreed Mum would have a tracheostomy. I felt that this was going to be the safest way to get her back to the UK on a medical plane that was being organised. I also felt that they were doing this as she was stable but that actually on returning to the UK the English doctors would start to prepare us to turn off the machine as ultimately Mum had made no progress.

However we arrived the next day to find Mum sitting up in bed with her eyes open and, although unable to really move, at least able to track with her eyes and follow us into the room! I grabbed Mum's hand and asked her to squeeze if she could hear me. I was absolutely stunned when she squeezed in response to this direct command and I have literally never felt so much hope come to me! I spent my allocated time trying to reassure Mum that she was safe and not to be scared, as people were looking after her. I just thought how scary it must be to be aware, as she was, and not be able to move.

At this point it was the end of my week's stay and I flew home with Sarah."

Josh

Josh waited for John's phone call, knowing that it was going to be about something important but he wasn't sure what it was most likely to be. When he was told he didn't think, at the time, it was going to be terribly serious in the long term. He knew I was currently in a coma but he had no further information. Straight away they decided to fly to Tenerife. Josh's main concern was for John as he felt how dreadful it must be for him coping with it all alone. He said it was great flying from Manchester because he could stay with his Aunty Sarah and her children. Josh is very fond of them and enjoyed being with them. Josh had trouble getting the time off work to visit Tenerife. His work said he wasn't able to have any compassionate leave but had to use his annual holiday. Josh also worried enormously that the news about me might appear on Facebook- in particular he feared that his work staff might refer to it on Facebook, not realising Sarah was away and that she might find out inappropriately.

Josh remembers a challenge at the airport as Roger had taken them to the wrong terminal and they had a last minute rush to find where to check in. He also found that lots of people asked him "Are you having a great holiday?" which was obviously not the case. When John met them at the airport he was pleased to be with his dad. Although he freely admits he would have liked to stay at home longer and tell Sarah the bad news he felt pleased to be there. He found the thought of visiting me difficult. However when he saw me he felt happier as he thought I just looked asleep. He liked Tenerife and enjoyed the museum trips and being with the family. When my Mum and Dad arrived he felt they should all stay together and that's why he tried to change his flight home. Josh thought the hospital was full of high-tech equipment and was confident that I was receiving the best possible care. However, apart from the reassurance that this was the case, he didn't feel that he received any support from hospital staff.

Josh became aware that I was paralysed down my right side. He hoped I would get well enough to be able to talk but didn't think I would ever walk or mobilise unaided. He left Tenerife with signs he might be right. In the future I might at least be well enough to talk!!

More from Hannah

Hannah and Josh were both distressed about leaving me. I had remained unconscious and, apart from moving my hand when James Blunt was played to my ear, there was no sign of any interaction or improvement. Hannah rang the flight company and asked them if it was possible to change the date of her flight home. She explained that her mum was unconscious and she wanted to stay with her. The woman who dealt with her didn't seem sympathetic at all and said it wasn't possible without further expense. In fact it was cheaper to fly home, buy another package holiday at home and come back to Tenerife later. So that's what Hannah reluctantly decided to do. It was their last day in Tenerife so it was arranged that they would visit me earlier, at lunch time visiting hours, so that they could get the coach to the airport later in the day.

When Hannah and Josh arrived at the intensive care unit for the last time they first waited at the end of the corridor. John went to speak to a doctor and Sarah came into my room. (There were strict rules that you could only visit in twos.) Hannah said it caused great distress to see Sarah pop into my room and quickly rush out. She wondered if the worst had happened. Sarah waved Hannah over and ran out so that Hannah could take her place. She rushed in and found, to her total amazement that I was off the ventilator, sitting up and appeared to be looking at her. She was totally amazed. I clearly looked poorly but I was alive!

Hannah recalls this being the best moment of her life. Her mum was clearly 'awake' and to her this was a very good sign for the future. However she was thinking that although I was alive I might not recover enough to actually speak to them or return to being the mother they knew. She noticed that I was looking around the room focusing on people. Hannah had read a little about spotting. This is when the person who has been unconscious focuses on you and appears to fix their gaze on you.

Hannah felt that it was unfair her brother and sisters were not sharing the exciting change. So she swapped with them. A short time later Josh and Hannah were in the room together. Josh made a joke and Hannah was sure that I had smiled, and she saw for the first time a face she knew. She explains how this smile was a facial expression that was just the kind of face I would have pulled at that joke had I been well. She thought this must be a good omen, although she had no medical information about what had happened. She guessed it was a good sign but she didn't know whether I might lapse back into unconsciousness. She had read that you can continue to recover for three years after a head injury. She thought, "If Mum has recovered so much after two weeks we don't know what will happen to her in three years' time."

The visiting hour finished and they had to leave. As their flight was not until later they all went to a restaurant. Hannah said there was a different mood. Although they were still very worried they now had a sense of hopefulness. Hannah and Sarah ordered a metre long sausage which was surprisingly cheap. This was the first time Hannah had let herself feel hope for the future- yet she still thought she would return to Tenerife. She remembers texting John's sister Sarah to tell her the good news.

The flight home felt very different from the flight out. On the way there she was preparing for death, thinking what she would feel like saying goodbye to her mum as 'a dead body'. Now she was flying back and her mother had just gained consciousness. It felt so different - still worrying, still scared, but in a nice way different.

She was excited in a way and really wanted to tell the world her mum had woken from her coma, but didn't feel it was appropriate to put the news on Facebook or anything as she still wasn't sure what this all meant. For example, was it possible that I might lapse back into a comatose state?

She usually waited for John or other family members to report updates before she spread any news and this time she didn't have to wait long. As they arrived back home she saw Josh had changed his status to 'Just got back from Tenerife with Hannah. Been visiting my mum who's been in a coma for the last twelve days, but on our very last visit Mum opened her eyes, squeezed my hand and even attempted to laugh at my terrible jokes! So very happy but a shame we had to fly home so soon after! Luckily she has her mum and dad out there to look after her now and we will see her again soon with Sarah, Charlotte & John!'

Hannah thought that this is just what she had been thinking, so she shared the status on her wall so that people knew the update.

They went back to John's sister's house to stay the night before returning home. It so happened that the Dunn family were on their way out to an Indian restaurant to celebrate a birthday so Hannah and Josh went with them. Hannah describes this as being really weird- she wanted to let herself celebrate but didn't know if she should yet. Sarah's family were really loud which is just like our family and Hannah remembers feeling very comfortable and welcome. The next day they were looking after their cousins and Sarah explained to the boys that we had come back from Tenerife as we had been visiting 'Auntie Kathy'. The eldest of the two boys, Kyan, said " Is Auntie Kathy in a poorly sleep?" Hannah thought that was a perfect description and smiled. She remembers thinking her five year old cousin had done a better job at telling her what was happening than the trained professionals at the hospital.

They then busied themselves making Get Well Soon cards:

CHAPTER EIGHT - JOHN'S STORY

It was day 2 of our cycle training camp. We had cycled to Puerto de Santiago and then completed a 20km climb up to Santiago del Teide which took us out of 24 degree sun and into rather cooler drizzle for the last few km. We then descended I think to Chio to wait for others including Kate, to rejoin. We stood back in the warm sun eating jelly babies and other energy boosters before we could all set off together for the remaining 20 km or so back to the hotel.

This was a long and fast descent and fairly quickly the group had split again as some of us went ahead learning how to take bends safely downhill (there's a lot more to it than you can imagine and it isn't intuitive!). However a small group of us stopped to wait for others to catch up. And wait. And wait. When you cycle ahead it can seem forever waiting for people but this was about 15 mins, so we decided to continue on in case they'd taken a different route. We got back to the hotel in Adeje and sat outside in glorious sun waiting for the others (we didn't have a key to the bike lockup!) A couple of other riders joined us and said they thought there'd been a puncture. But eventually we had probably been waiting anything up to an hour. We heard ambulances in the distance. Someone's phone rang. A shocked facial expression - was that a glance at me? Then I was passed the phone.

I was told that there'd been an accident - no cars involved. Ambulances were present and Kate was going to be taken straight to hospital. I was to be taken to the scene of the accident and someone else would look after my bike and belongings.

The location was a quiet, wide and straight road running near a golf course. The road was closed off and half way down there was an ambulance and police were photographing the scene. Near the ambulance Kate's bike stood against a fence - one shoe still attached. A few of her belongings were on the road - including her smashed cycling goggles. I walked over to the rear of the ambulance and called, "Kathy". A paramedic appeared, indicated 'no' and put his finger to his lips. The door, I recall, was then closed - was that a drip?

I was taken back to the hotel as the ambulance drove away. I was being looked after by Jeanette, one of the leaders. They had things planned. I was to get a bag of belongings and they would then drive me to the hospital - about 75km away in Santa Cruz, that's the other end of the island! (I thought I had done this quite well - choosing some clothes that would be comfortable in bed, and a set for returning to the hotel, underwear, shoes ... all for Kathy. I hadn't realised that these were meant to be for me). The journey to the hospital de la Candelaria in Santa Cruz seemed to take for hours. I cannot recall a thing. I sat nervously in silence with a sense of guilt that yet again I had cycled on ahead without waiting for Kate.

The area around the hospital seemed to be like a building site. There were no parking spaces so cars double parked and you gave your key to a stranger in a yellow cycling vest so that he could move the car into a space or out of the way of someone trying to leave!!

We were asked to sit in a waiting room next to A&E - unpleasant, crowded, noisy - probably for an hour, maybe two. We spoke to a doctor who had invited us into an office. It was a serious trauma to the head. It was very serious, "I am sorry, but it is very bad". Kate was currently with doctors who were assessing her. When they could they'd take us to see her. More waiting, now upstairs in a waiting room next to Intensive Care. How many hours? How long since the accident? 5 hours maybe?

Jeanette had put some pieces of the puzzle together, but none was for sure.

The remaining four cyclists were spread out in single file down the road when there was the awful sound of a crash behind. The second cyclist put his brakes on shouting 'stopping' to see what had happened. The third cyclist turned around causing her to crash into the second cyclist. This resulted in concussion and broken bones. The second cyclist, one of the leaders, had a dilemma - who should he deal with? Kate was some way away and appeared to be sat up. He attended to the cyclist who had crashed into him. He sent the first cyclist, who returned from further down the road after a minute or two, up to support Kate. This was probably traumatic for him - Kate was suffering from facial injuries and passed into unconsciousness. What had caused the crash? No one will know. Kate crashed next to an exit from a golf course. The police had wondered if a golf buggy may have started to exit, caused the crash, and quickly turned back. But there is no evidence for this. There was, however, a speed ramp. A short sharp bump up and then a 'platform' before a bump back down maybe 5 metres later. It was innocuous - but if Kate hadn't seen it? I have seen cyclists crash before when they hit a bump they are not expecting. I have unexpectedly seen a bump too late after I have involuntarily let go of the handle bars, planted my private parts on the cross bar and spent about 5 seconds careering down a road with the bike snaking beneath me before regaining control!

We were then called down to intensive care. A long corridor with short bays going off to the right, each one with just 3 or 4 beds in their own room. I was told that the doctor could see me now and to go to the room at the end. I walked down with Jeanette following (she had asked me what I wanted and I asked if she would mind coming with me so that she could hear what was said more objectively.) We walked into the room. No doctor, just a patient propped in a bed. Their head was clean-shaven. Tubes appeared to protrude from all parts of the body - including the head. There were swabs covering some facial injuries. The white sheets were pristine. The head appeared swollen - out of proportion. How long did it take until I realised it was Kate? I felt Jeanette's hand on my shoulder. I could hear my pulse beating in my head.

A doctor did come to talk - he had limited English and took us to an office with another member of staff whose English was a little better. Severe traumatic brain injury. Coma. No responses. Scans showed deep lacerations to the brain and not isolated but in many parts of the brain. The wounds on the face are not treated yet as they await a plastic surgeon to make a professional job. They could not say if she would survive but repeated that it was very severe. The next few hours or days would be crucial.

I kissed Kate on the hand and stroked her cheek. I whispered that I loved her and I said, "Take your time. You will be OK, don't fight now, save your energy". If she could hear I didn't want her to worry about me, but to focus on recovering however well she could - I told her this.

Jeanette had everything planned. They had a property about half way between the hospital and the hotel. They would take me to stay with them and not return to the hotel ... Oh, and they had dogs. The sort that gang together to eat you once the owners are out of sight (she didn't say this). On the journey to their house I sobbed. Strange how easy that became over the next few days that I stayed with them - sometimes Jeanette would cry with me - which was worrying as she was usually driving at the time.

From that base we could visit Kate over the next few days. I could contemplate life, think about plans of action, and cry myself to sleep. I needed to think about who to tell, when and why. It would be the children first - they are adults. Sarah, 16, was the youngest and skiing with school. I didn't want her hearing accidentally, perhaps through Facebook - and I didn't want a 'stranger' telling her. I also wanted her to finish her holiday and then be back home with the support of her siblings around her. It is now Tuesday and she is back on Saturday. I wanted to tell the other three but in a situation where they were not alone either - Wednesday would be best. By then I may have a clearer prognosis about Kathy.

These few days were lived in a bit of a protective daze. The only task I completed was to contact the insurers. I did look after the dogs for a while. They were getting very boisterous. Probably only play but at one point one puppy seemed to be getting hurt and there was barking and squealing. I shouted "Stop" and was impressed to see that they stopped in their tracks. I was slightly less impressed at the menacing stare that they all gave me for the next few minutes!

Visiting times were very limited. The impression I have of Spanish healthcare? Outstanding care for the patient ... possibly less time for the relatives - but with no Spanish at all perhaps I was missing something. So 1pm doctor time (20 mins or so when a specialist may be able to update you). 7pm visiting for up to an hour, max 2 at a time…. I think.

There was no progress with Kate. Scans, drugs, responses ... nothing was good. The specialists were mainly trying to stabilise the situation and it was still too early to know exactly how Kate would progress ... but they repeated how poor things seemed to be. Kate's head was shaved in case there was a need for brain surgery or to drill into the skull to reduce pressure on the brain. They were hoping not to have to do this.

The accident had happened on Monday. It was now Wednesday and really Kate's condition had not changed. Although she had not deteriorated I got the impression that the lack of response was not good. They had discovered that she responded to pain on her left side but that she was totally paralysed on her right side. Numerous tubes were attached, either ventilating her, feeding her or administering medication.

Today I would tell Charlotte, Hannah and Josh and ask them not to tell Sarah until she is back home safe from her ski trip - they would look after each other.

I would need to impress on them the seriousness of Kathy's condition, that any change in her, positive or negative, is likely to be over weeks or months. They would not be able to share information on social media until Sarah was home. I would take responsibility for letting Janet and Bernard know but nobody else could know until Sarah is home ... All assuming I and they could handle the call!

And how do you make 3 calls at the same time? There was just a chance that Charlotte would be at home - she was regularly home on Wednesdays for Netball. I called her during the afternoon - she was at the local garden centre with her fiancé and agreed to drive straight home so that I could call her and Josh (it transpired that she thought either I had broken my leg or 'mum' was pregnant!). Whilst she was driving home I phoned Hannah.

I won't go in to a lot of detail about the calls. Having attempted to explain it all without becoming emotional, and failing, I tried to tell them not to fly out. They needed to support Sarah and each other - and then fly out when things got a little clearer.

The next I knew Hannah and Josh were booked on a flight out and Charlotte would follow with Sarah on Sunday!

Quick chronology

Monday 18th Feb
Accident approximately 2pm.

Unseen as she was the last rider in a group of four, about 25m back. Appears to have crashed at a speed bump, just at entrance to golf course. Noise of crash appears to have caused two riders ahead to collide and crash and one of these was taken to hospital in a separate ambulance. The two remaining riders attended to the victims. Kate appears to have landed on her face (right side) as minor damage to front/edge of helmet. No pedestrians or other vehicles in the vicinity. Police closed the road and two ambulances attended.

Taken to Candelaria Hospital, sedated, about an hour or more later, after stabilising at roadside. Visited hospital about 5pm. Advised of serious bleeding to the brain, cuts/damage to the face. CT scan revealed no other damage to the rest of the body. One side of body (right side if I recall and possibly just arm) not responding to pain.

Around 10pm allowed to see Kate, she was sedated/unconscious. Doctor reiterated the information above. Also explained that they were sedating etc and for short periods reducing this to check for response. Did not expect to have a true picture for 48 hrs.

Moved in with Jen, Stuart and 3 dogs.

Tuesday 19th

Hired car to travel to hospital / hotel etc. Collected belongings. Visited hospital at 1pm. Allowed to see Kate. Condition no change. Advised by doctor that she would have another CT scan and we may have more information at 1pm tomorrow. Talking of serious brain damage.

Around 4pm advised insurers of the incident. 5.30 pm (approx) forms were completed, scanned and returned to insurers.

Money problem. I can't access Kate's account to manage her money and transfer money due into my account. I know the password but not the security question!

Wed/Thurs 20/21 Feb

Visits on both days. No change to Kate's condition. Received a call from the insurers' Doctor to confirm Kate's status. Detailed report confirming all above and advising they expect a clearer picture next week and will call on Monday.

Wed pm.
Called Hannah and Charlotte/Josh to give them the news then phoned Bernard. We will keep from Sarah until she gets back on Saturday.

Thursday
Told a few other close friends by email, also Kate's PA and my Headteacher.

Friday 22nd Feb
Josh and Hannah arrived in Tenerife. I moved into a hotel with them in Santa Cruz (Adonis Plaza). Close to tram that goes to hospital. Visited Kate in the evening. Sedation may be reduced. Having told J & H that Kate is motionless apart from her relaxed breathing, she appeared to shake her legs slightly. At one point she yawned and opened her eyes. Brought tears to my eyes (again). (Do seem to have developed a problem with my tear ducts ... they seem to have developed a continuous leak)

Saturday 23rd Feb
Visited again but no Doctor (we are happy to get a fuller up-date on Monday). Kate seemed even more restless. She was stretching her whole body with arms and legs stretching towards her feet. She even seemed to move her right arm. Her legs also bent at the knee and kicked out a little. Injuries to face healing a little.

Sarah met by Charlotte from Ski trip with school. Spoke on phone with Sarah, who sounded far too sensible like the others had. They are both flying out tomorrow. Hotel just 100m away from ours (Hotel Atlantique).

Sunday 24th Feb

Money problem. The expected pin didn't work on the cash passport so I now can't get out our 'holiday' Euros.

Visited Kate. Still lots of movement from her but her level of breathing was scary, as though she was fighting the ventilator. Josh, Hannah and I talking to her in case she can hear us. Her movements might have indicated she can?

Met Charlotte and Sarah at north airport, minus their baggage lost in transit by the operator. Then their hotel was poor. Then Sarah got upset as I talked to her about Mum, in MacDonald's.

Monday 25th Feb

Charlotte's bag delivered ... Sarah's bag still missing.

Kate's condition appears stable. Little progress though. Eye movement, some leg movement ... Not enough. Kids very good talking to her, letting her know they are there.

Tuesday 26th Feb

Doctor confirmed all that we know. Also that the pressure on the brain is now OK, which we suspected. However, she is no longer sedated and they were hoping that she would respond to some instructions like squeeze my finger, which she hasn't. They reiterated that the process is going to be very slow. They also requested my consent for a tracheostomy.

Weds 27th Feb

Signed consent for tracheostomy. Kate making some new movement with her left arm, in towards centre line. Some very small responses to our presence. I asked insurers about repatriation. They feel that the tracheostomy will further stabilise her condition and they can then begin to assess the possibility of an air ambulance.

Thursday 28th Feb

Kate serene (on morphine). Tracheostomy has been successful and we can now see how well her facial injuries are healing. She looks beautiful and very young! Little response today though.

Friday 1st March

What a day. Exhausted. Josh and Hannah checked out and we all went to visit Kate, 'en route to the airport'. We were amazed. She had her eyes open, though not well focused. She squeezed my hand on request. She smiled when she obtained eye contact with me and I was smiling at her. It was astounding progress. It doesn't tell us how far she will progress, but it was an astonishing leap forward. It made it very difficult for Hannah and Josh to leave. We went for a slap up meal to celebrate before they left.

It wasn't long before Sarah, Charlotte and I met Janet and Bernard on the tram to the hospital. It was a good first visit for them. Kate tired but similar to lunchtime. It was a surprise for them. It was a great day for Kate.

Weekend 2/3rd March

We visited twice on Saturday but Kate was asleep on both occasions. Each visit though we notice slight developments but she was still on morphine so we forgave her the sleeping! Sunday we had a lousy journey home.

Over the next few days communicating with people on the phone, via email and then through Facebook became a full time job. So I have included some of the emails in a final chapter and indicated who I was communicating with.

CHAPTER NINE
MY PARENTS' STORIES

BERNARD:

It was a Wednesday in mid February. We had booked a day trip by ship to France, and had invited our friend Mary to come with us. We had a lovely day, it was sunny and mild, and as well as a good meal, we had had an interesting walk round an old fortified town just east of Calais. We were on our way back on the ferry when I received a strange text message. I say "strange" because it was from Kathy's phone, but was signed from John. He asked "Where are you? I've been trying to ring you."

Janet was immediately concerned. She said that she knew that Kathy and John were in Tenerife, and that we had not heard from them as was usually the case. So I tried to ring Kathy's phone, but without success.

A little later, still before we docked, there was another message. This time from Josh who wrote "Dad is trying to contact you!" As soon as we got ashore, I stopped in a lay-by and rang Josh. He repeated that John needed to talk to us. I said "Is it something serious?" and he replied "Yes, very!" I felt that it would be wrong to ask him for further details, and that I should try to get in touch with John, so we drove on home.

As soon as we got home I rang Kathy's phone. John answered and told me that there had been an accident on Monday, that Kathy was in IT in a hospital in Santa Cruz, and that she was in a coma. Janet was standing near me trying to read my face and guess what was being said. John filled me in with the main details of what had happened, and we agreed to keep in touch by email as it was difficult for us both to talk, both being overwhelmed by the situation.

John had reminded us that Sarah was on a skiing holiday, and so it would be sensible to keep the news among ourselves until she returned on Saturday and someone could explain everything to her. We couldn't have her continuing with her holiday while worrying about her Mum's condition. So we rang Alan and close relatives and repeated the need to keep things quiet for the time being.

The next few days were very difficult. We were in touch with our four grandchildren, discussing who should fly out to Tenerife and when. It was decided that Josh and Hannah should go as soon as possible, and that Charlotte would meet Sarah off the school bus when she returned from holiday, and break the news to her. They would then fly out the following day. That left us to start making our own arrangements. One complication was that Janet had eye injections coming up early in March which she could not miss. So I booked a return flight for her, and just a single for myself. This was to be for the following weekend, just before John was due to return himself.

How we got through those days I shall never know. It all seems like a nightmare now. We had to make plans, but people were helpful in offering transport and other help. News seemed so scarce, I do remember being told that Kathy's unconscious state was probably because she was in an induced coma. However a day or two later we heard that this was no longer the case, but that she was still unconscious. I was desperate. I felt that the one thing that I could cling onto for hope had just been pulled away from me. We were in Waitrose, and I stumbled along the aisles my eyes full of tears. It seemed that by the time we got to the hospital, my daughter might be already dead. I tried to think of what I would say at the funeral, and whether I could handle it. I felt that I would have to be strong for the sake of the grandchildren, and of course for John and my wife Janet, but I doubted whether I could do it.

As it got nearer to departure day, things were a little easier because there was so much arranging to be done. Getting insurance because I was now 80 and no longer automatically covered for example. There simply wasn't time to think about the awful possibilities of what might yet happen. Alan drove us to Gatwick, and we joined a crowd of excited youngsters going off for a holiday in the sun. People asked us where we were going and what we were planning to do, and we had to tell them the truth which of course made them embarrassed and they probably regretted having spoken to us!

When we arrived at Tenerife, we were expecting to see Josh and Hannah who were just on their way back to England. There was no sign of them at the airport, and I rang John's phone to see if any meeting place had been arranged. In my confused state, I had rung John's Dad (also called John), and he tried to calm me down while I tried to get rid of him so that I could concentrate on finding the grandchildren. I still feel bad about the way I spoke to him!

It soon became obvious that we weren't going to see Josh and Hannah, so we bought tickets and found the bus to Santa Cruz. When we arrived at the bus station, John rang to say that if we got on a tram immediately, they would join us in a couple of stops and we could go to the hospital with them. I pointed out that we had all our luggage with us, but John said that wouldn't matter, and a few minutes later there they were getting on our tram. They were all smiles and obviously pleased to see us, but I was puzzled that they seemed so upbeat considering why we were all here at all! However, it soon became obvious that there was better news about Kathy, she had made some kind of contact with them, however brief, and they felt that whatever the outcome, she wasn't going to die.

I can't convey what relief this brought to me, and I eagerly looked forward to getting off the tram and seeing her for myself. But all was not to be so straightforward. It was raining hard, and the temporary path to the hospital entrance was steeply downhill. I was pulling a large heavy case on wheels, and the slope caused it to gather speed and knock me off my feet. I went down with a sickening thud onto the hard concrete. For a moment I thought that I was going to be in a hospital bed too. I think that John, who was in front, had helped to break my fall, and although bruised and painful, I was able to be helped to my feet, relieved of my luggage, and escorted into the hospital waiting room.

John explained where we had to go and where we had to wait, and realising we were going to have to do this for ourselves soon, I tried to take it all in. After quite a long wait, we were taken to the IC unit. Only two at a time were allowed to enter the bay where each patient lay, and I let Janet go first, I'm not sure who went with her. When it was my turn, I was shocked with what I saw. I simply couldn't recognise this person lying there as my Kathryn. Her head was shaved, she had tubes and wires going in and out of every orifice, and she just lay inert without giving a sign of life. If it hadn't been for the good news that we had learned in the tram, I would have given up hope there and then.

Looking back now, nearly two years later, I find it hard to recall the exact sequence of events. However I did write daily emails, particularly to John, Kate's husband, and these have been included in his account. I will let these emails tell the story of that week in Tenerife.

At the end of the year, Kathy gave us a Kent calendar, and suggested that we should meet every month at the place pictured. We have done that now thirteen times, and I've no doubt we will continue with this arrangement until we are too disabled to do it any more. This is one of the more positive outcomes of Kathy's accident. We all realise how fragile life is, and how much we value and love each other. We are so close now, and that's the way it's going to remain!

JANET:

On the morning of 8th March I was up early. We'd been staying in Tenerife for six days because we had to fly out to see our daughter Kathryn, who, as you know had been seriously injured in a bicycle accident. We were up early because the Insurance Company had arranged a flight home to England for that day. We had been told that we had to report to the hospital at 6.30am. We arrived early, but were anxious because the hospital was not open to visitors and security would not allow us in. However our taxi driver seeing our plight phoned our hotel and the receptionist explained to him that we would be able to enter at 6.30am. This was all done with some difficulty due to our lack of Spanish. On entering the hospital and finding our way to the ward some few minutes later we found Katie having her breakfast. That is, if you think of breakfast as a bowlful of gruel. This was given to her by a nurse. She wasn't able to feed herself.

Not long after the Doctor and the Nurse from the air ambulance arrived. We had met them briefly the previous evening just before we had left from our daily visit. They went off to complete the formalities of handing over a patient and I was urged to visit the toilet as there was no toilet on board the aircraft.

Sometime later, in a procession we made our way through the labyrinth of corridors to the exit of the hospital where an ambulance was waiting. I said goodbye to Bernard, my husband, who was not allowed to come with us. I went in the back of the ambulance with Katie and the Nurse. It was not a comfortable ride at all but fortunately not too long a journey.

When we arrived at the airport we were taken to a part of the complex where special assignments were taken, not the part of the airport where tourists normally go. I was asked to get out and was given back my passport which had been in the care of the nurse. I was taken to a shed like place where I was asked to show my passport. And I have a feeling that I probably also had to be searched but part of it is a little bit hazy to me but I do remember trying to explain that I had a new hip which sets the alarm off.

Then I rejoined the ambulance crew and the Doctor and the Nurse and we were taken out onto the runway where the plane was waiting for us. It was an extremely small aeroplane that was fit for the purpose. When we entered the plane Katie was put from the stretcher onto a special bed. There was a lot of equipment around. The plane was basically like this:- on the left hand side were three seats, two facing each other, and one single. On the other side were the two stretcher-like beds, the one towards the back of the plane was the one Kathryn was put on. Underneath the bed there was medical equipment with wires and dials. As there was only one patient, I think the other stretcher was used for the food which the pilots and the doctor and nurse brought with them in cold boxes for us all. Then there was just the tail of the plane which was used for other medical equipment and my very small case. Of course the two pilots were in the cockpit at the front.

Soon afterwards we took off and the Nurse pointed out the mountain she could see with snow on it. I have to say I didn't actually see that. I could see the coastline as we flew out over Tenerife. The doctor told me we would be two hours before we stopped again but in fact I think it was nearly four. As we approached a seaside place with beaches and houses on either side, I had absolutely no idea where we were.

We landed and the Nurse and I left Kathryn in the hands of the doctor and the two pilots and we were driven out in a very posh Mercedes across the runway to some buildings where there were very nice toilets which were most welcome. We were watched most of the time, I think for security. It reminded me a little bit of a James Bond film with a man standing in a very posh black overcoat and directing all the proceedings. The man spoke English, and I asked where we were and he told me it was where port wine came from - Oporto in Portugal. While the plane was being refuelled the three men were taken to the toilet and then it was time to set off again.

I felt more relaxed and Katie seemed fine and sometimes tried to talk. The Nurse and I took turns to sit close to her, but mostly she slept. At one time she was given something to eat and drink (contents of the cold box seemed to cover all eventualities) which caused some consternation as she began to splutter. Then she was put on a machine, I think to clear her, and the doctor seemed satisfied that the fluid had been removed from her lungs. She seemed to know we were there but we had to keep an eye on her because she kept undoing her seat belt. This was important because she was lying on a kind of large baby changing mat which had sides but would not have kept her from falling off if the plane had lurched. We joked that she was a naughty girl but in truth it was a most welcome sign because in order to do this she had to use both hands and there had been concern that her right side had been affected.

Towards the end of the afternoon when it was beginning to get dark I noticed that we were flying over some small buildings, or at least they seemed small, and soon we had landed at Biggin Hill. It was quite a relief to know that we were back in England and that she was safe. An ambulance was supposed to be waiting for us but it hadn't arrived and as it was cold and not very pleasant with the door of the plane open, we were pushed into a very, very large hangar where we waited. The Doctor, Nurse and Pilots went off and tried to negotiate our departure.

Eventually the ambulance arrived. Katie was taken from the plane at four pm to the back of the ambulance and I was just about to go in too as I had done in Tenerife when I was told "No, you have got to sit at the front as she is going to be well looked after with a paramedic, doctor and a nurse and there isn't room for you." As I was trying to put my seatbelt on, the driver gave me a little talk. He said "I want you to relax. I don't want you to react to anything I do. Today you will go on a journey that I hope you will not have to do again."

The journey was, I have to say, rather exciting because it was on full alert with lights flashing and sirens blaring. People were very responsive, making as much room as possible, and I found myself wanting to acknowledge their efforts. By this time, it was getting darker, it was raining and rather misty.

Arriving at Maidstone Hospital, there was some delay as decisions had to be made about where to take Kate. Eventually she was taken into a ward, lifted from the stretcher and placed on a bed. Although she had spoken little previously, she noticed an old lady in a bed opposite and enquired in a husky voice, "Is she all right?" It seemed to me that she was beginning to be the Nurse again and that was a good sign.

By this time John had found us in the hospital and was reunited with Katie. This was a great relief to me as when, a couple of days previously, I had told her we were flying home to find John she had wrinkled up her nose and I was fearful she might not recognise him. However I need not have worried.

The Nurse on the ward offered Katie a cup of tea and I became agitated because to my knowledge she had not drunk from a cup since her accident. I also remembered the incident in the plane!! However I explained this to John and between us we alerted the staff. I did find it hard to explain, though, as I couldn't think on the spur of the moment the name of the apparatus that had previously been used.

By this time the Doctor and the Nurse had returned to Biggin Hill but I don't know if the ambulance took them or whether they had a taxi. I do know that Vikki the Nurse was hoping to go out for a meal that evening in Exeter!!

I was taken to Kathy's home but John stayed behind at the hospital. Alan our son picked me up on his way home to Wye where he was living at that time. Cheryl had prepared a delicious chicken meal. This was most welcome as I had had very little to eat all day.

At the end of the day I felt a little lost because suddenly I was no longer with Katie. And after such a busy day although tired I couldn't sleep so wrote the next verse of my poem.

Kate has asked me to say something of how I felt about this memorable day. Usually I am very uneasy about hospitals and people being ill, as I am not sure how to react. However I had had five days with Katie, had seen her first signs of recovery, had got used to seeing her without hair and realised that she had recognised her father and me. Once she was moved to a ward we had spent many hours with her. The difficult time was when we left her because she looked so vulnerable in a room all on her own. It reminded us of when she was one year old and taken to hospital with gastroenteritis. In those days parents were not allowed to stay with their children and the atmosphere was very austere. So those feelings of protectiveness came to the fore once more and although of course we talked to her as an adult, joked etc, played music on our visits, I felt uneasy when we had to leave her, as we had done when she was little.

Perhaps too on the journey, although very involved, I was not responsible for any of the decisions and that made it easier for me. I remember walking down the corridor at

Maidstone Hospital with the stretcher and its entourage and noticing people passing by and thinking that normally I would be upset by such a sight, but on this occasion we were talking and behaving as if it was quite a natural thing. I think when we are faced with difficult situations we are given strength to manage. When Kathryn was in intensive care and just beginning to make sense of the world the Nurse approached me and asked if I would feed her because he said "She won't open her mouth for me". For a moment I panicked. It was the last thing I expected. I rushed to disinfect my hands at the end of the ward and went back to the cubicle to start choosing the food. There was an array of tubs with various semi-liquid foods but I chose yoghurt which was familiar. We both encouraged her to take it and the male nurse was really pleased with our success.

All these incidents have brought us much closer together and it has been a privilege to be part of her recovery.

JANET'S POEM

Today I need to speak to God
About our daughter Kate
She's fallen from her bicycle
She is in a serious state
No longer can she speak or hear, ignoring those around.
Recovery will be long, we're told, before we hear a sound
So please God, help us be brave, awaiting for her voice
And bring her back to normal life
And then we can rejoice!

Friday 8th March 2013

Today as planned, I'll talk to God
About our daughter Kate
With grateful heart, our hopes now high,
This news we can relate.
She now is able to mouth to us
And listen to our talk
She moves a lot and wants to eat
One day we hope she'll walk.
Today we brought her back to Kent
Where she'll recuperate.
Her friends and family all join
To thank you, God, for Kate.

Wednesday 27th March 2013

Today, with thanks, I'll speak to God
About our daughter Kate.
Her progress good, I'm glad to say,
She'll do well at this rate.
Now she can speak and read her cards,
Friends she can recognise.
She's walking well, goes to the gym
Where she can exercise.
Her brain at present needs must rest,
Forgets from day-to-day.
She gets confused but knows she is,
While nature takes its way.
Allowed home for weekend break
With all else left behind,
On Monday off to Sevenoaks
Where specialist help she'll find.

April 2013

Today again I'll speak to God
About our daughter Kate
She's doing well at Sevenoaks,
We know this news is great.
She's learning how to cope with life,
Facing the world around.
Coming to terms with her accident
Is difficult, she's found.
She's willing to stay for four more weeks
To get the help that's best.
Although the clock goes slowly,
It gives her time to rest.
Beginning now to do some chores,
She's able to bake a cake.
She potters round and sees TV
And calls to friends can make.
To see her now, so very well,
We can't believe it is true!
So grateful are we for her life
We have to say "thank-you.

June 2013

Today I'd like to talk to God
About our daughter Kate.
It's four months since her accident,
The progress made is great!
She now can cope with many things,
Loves friends and family,
Rides tandem on her husband's bike,
Her fitness is the key!
The future still is not too clear
About her post as Head.
But never mind the outcome,
She'll be content, she said.
So once again our heartfelt thanks
For giving Kate her life,
To live it to the full again
As mother, daughter, wife.

CHAPTER TEN – BACK IN ENGLAND
WHAT DO I REMEMBER?

Clearly the family were keen for me to be back in England but the children were very worried about how I would be on my return. They felt they had not seen me for a long time and had been relying on other people for information about my progress.

They realised that I would have a very poor memory, and Hannah was particularly concerned that I wouldn't recognize them. Hannah just couldn't stop thinking about what it would be like if her mum didn't know who she was, and how she would cope with something like this. Hannah remembers,

'I was so eager to get to the hospital to see what she could remember and most importantly who she could remember. We were all by her hospital bed and mum looked at us all and smiled a confused smile. My heart sank. She then proceeded to speak... "Charlotte, Hannah, Joshua"... as if she knew what had been worrying us. Then there was a long pause before finally she said.... "Sarah."

She had named us all in age order! Which was actually quite impressive as most of what else came out of her mouth that day and for months after made absolutely no sense at all. She didn't recognise most people who were not in the immediate family. She used very strange words. I knew not to just pretend I understood what she was talking about, so we would just say: I am not sure what you mean.

I remember for quite a while Mum would get completely the wrong word for things, so she would ask Dad to get food out of the washing machine, when really she was asking for plates out of the dishwasher - Dad would get an earful when he went looking in the washing machine! She also answered questions quite wrongly, for example telling people that she took sugar in her tea when that was not the case, or saying that her favourite sport was ballet when she had never done ballet but was a keen cyclist.

Another example of her memory problems concerned passwords. Dad was keen to change their bank details so that he could check all the finances were in order but although Mum told him quite confidently what her password was, it proved to be wrong and Dad could not access the bank account. After she was allowed home for a short time before going to rehab Dad took Mum to the bank, explained the situation and the bank took Mum into a room to change the password securely. Dad wasn't sure Mum would remember but the bank insisted Mum had to be on her own. Of course when Mum got out and Dad asked for the password, she had no idea what it was.

Mum became very sad as she started to gain more awareness. She felt she was being judged all the time and didn't trust anyone outside the family (which is difficult as she was being cared for in a rehab unit). I was trying to think of things to cheer her up and had the idea of contacting a few celebrities to see if they would wish her well. To my surprise the cyclist Chris Hoy responded to my tweet, wishing her a speedy recovery. I hope this helped!'

So what do I remember about the whole incident? To be honest, very little. I don't remember anything about Tenerife or my three week stay in hospital there. I find that really sad – the fact that staff worked hard, saved my life and yet haven't been thanked by me appropriately. I have sent a thank you letter to staff at the hospital as well as the paramedics who presumably did literally save my life at the roadside. As yet I don't know if they have ever received my thank you. I so want that to happen. I have some memories but think some of them are inaccurate, for example being in a plane, flying home, and going inside a building for plane maintenance work. I am sure that is unlikely to have happened. I remember a trip out of Maidstone Hospital for a visit to a chip shop near the hospital grounds. Charlotte has told me that this did happen - she took me one day towards the end of my stay at the hospital but I remember thinking at the time it was a dream and not happening in reality. It seems that some work colleagues and friends visited me while in Maidstone hospital but I remember very little of this, only being told they had come in the months that followed.

I was weak and had lost weight. I remember getting on the scales at home and being 7.5 stone. Everyone who saw me in hospital says that I actually hated it. I am sure the staff were good but I am told I watched everything that was done and criticised the care patients were receiving. I was holding on to my nurse management role without the authority, knowledge or skills to do so and now guess I was a complete nightmare to look after. I have no knowledge to back my view that care was substandard but I was confused and not functioning normally and that is what I was thinking at the time. I would love to tell you that I actually remember the care I received being rather good but sadly I don't remember it either way at all. However John would have dealt with poor care and Charlotte my nurse daughter would have noticed if things were poor and would have dealt with any concerns they might have had. So I am guessing now it was fine.

However there is one incident which I think actually happened but which may only be a memory of a dream. Nursing staff were giving me a bed bath. The nurses were talking to each other about their night out the previous evening and they did not once speak to me as they rolled me over to wash me. In fact they started talking together about intimate details of their relationships, including whether to sleep with their newly acquired partners or not.

Whilst I have no idea if this actually happened I feel deep down that it did. I just want to take this opportunity to say to care staff who might be in this position, "Would you like it? Speak to the client even if they can't talk back. Treat them as individuals, as humans deserving of respect. Just because they can't respond don't treat them badly. Would you talk about your sex life to a 51 year old woman who you don't know well? Of course not, so don't do it to me, or anyone else who can't respond."

After a while I was transferred from Maidstone to the rehabilitation unit in Sevenoaks. I really didn't want to go there. Charlotte said it was clear I just wanted to be at home. John found it difficult. The medical staff felt I would be better with good rehabilitation and John said that when they actually talked to me about its benefits I did agree to this but the minute their backs were turned I was vocal to everyone about not wanting to go. It seemed my head injury had stopped me behaving appropriately. I was a different person.

In the end I agreed to go because I felt it would enable John to go to work and I could be cared for whilst he was out. I didn't feel the unit had any benefits for me personally. John clearly has another viewpoint and feels the unit helped me move forward. The staff were professional and I recognize that they worked hard to accommodate my needs. I hated being there, though, and became aware that I was clinically depressed. I have never suffered from a depressive disorder so I had no reference points. However I woke every day feeling that pleasurable life had ended. Suicide was on my list to do if I could do it and ensure my children weren't damaged in any way. My memory was bad and I wasn't sure of simple facts like who the prime minister was. I was aware that this was highly abnormal and would mean my career was at risk. Being in the middle ground, not knowing or being able to do something, but being totally aware that I used to do it, and should be able to do it, was extremely depressing. I felt that it would be better for everyone if I just died. Clearly I didn't want to upset my family and I realised that they were actually feeling more positive about my health. However I was on the way down, thinking things were worse for me.

So I went home for a weekend and then on Monday morning I set off with John to Sevenoaks rehabilitation unit. The weekend at home had been great. John's sister Sarah had come to stay with her children and Johnny, John's brother. I have a partial recollection of the weekend. I remember feeling a fraud that I didn't feel unwell and I was going for a long hospital stay. What would people think of me? Surely I could look after myself at home? My hospital reports say I was very unstable and likely to fall but I didn't realise this. I know I slept a little during the day but otherwise had no understanding that I wasn't behaving normally.

I am told that I repeated conversations when speaking. I know we all do this a bit but I am told I did it constantly for 18 months. It still happens but less often.

I remember the weekend before my admission to Sevenoaks but I don't remember being admitted. John was struggling. He had been told by medical staff that I needed to be there but I really didn't feel I needed it. I hated being watched. With my damaged mind I felt that I was being judged as to whether I was a nice person or not. When I didn't do well at cognitive tests I thought it was proof that I was hopeless and therefore needed to commit suicide to free the world of a hopeless case. Because of this I refused to take part in the testing and I had a sense that again I was being naughty not participating according to the plan. I want to say the staff made it bearable but only just - suicide was a constant thought. I woke up thinking about it and thought it right through the day until bedtime.

The only thing that stopped me doing something dramatic was my lovely family, but one day even that wasn't enough. My blood pressure had risen a bit and so I decided that I was too hard work for my family to care for anymore. I thought I would ring the children and tell them that although I loved them I also realised that my time had come to an end. I loved them so much but in time they would get on with their lives and not have a mother to care for. I rang Hannah and started to tell her. Clearly the conversation was difficult and she tried to tell me that it wasn't a good idea. However as I put the phone down I had a sense of normal thinking. Why had I done that and upset my lovely daughter? The medics had been persuading me to start antidepressants. I had constantly re-fused them but as I put the phone down I wondered if they might help my despair. I hadn't believed antidepressants could help. I was depressed in my mind because I had had an accident and now in my mind I was no longer normal and so life was not worth living. That is what the problem was - I wasn't normal anymore and I didn't like it. I so wanted to behave and think normally and I didn't feel antidepressants could help with that.

As I read this I realise how badly my brain was dam-aged. I am a strong advocate of people's rights if they have a disability of any type. I have a lot of patience and understand-ing especially with those that have a learning disability. I believe strongly that we all have a right, if we are disabled, to live a full life and for our disabilities to be accepted and compensated for by others. The only person I had no tolerance for was myself. When I put the phone down, after speaking to Hannah, I had a sense I was being unfair. I wondered whether I should at least try antidepressants. I went and found a nurse to discuss the matter and started them the next day.

There were many examples of good care at Sevenoaks rehabilitation unit. In particular my key worker persuaded me that staying would help and she was nice. In a different situation she could have been a friend and so I agreed to stay for six weeks. All other patients stayed for months so six weeks seemed bearable, although not in any way pleasant. So that is what I agreed to. I felt it was slowing down my recovery and I wanted to plan and deliver this myself. I appreciate that I was ill and this may have altered my perception but I am telling you what I felt at the time. However I do feel, even now, that if somebody has had a head injury it is assumed that what they say doesn't make sense. So when I gave my view about anything it was often not regarded as appropriate. It was hard to move from running an organisation to my current state, with nobody really valuing what I thought or said. I held this view for a long period of time and sadly still do at times with certain people.

My mum and dad came to see me in Sevenoaks and I remember thinking they should be told I have had an accident but things are looking OK. I planned to tell them this and was completely unaware that they had actually been to Tenerife and my mum had flown back with me. I don't remember being told what had happened - I just slowly picked it up over many months.

My right arm hurt me and I wasn't able to move it. Charlotte told me that I had been paralysed down my right side and didn't move anything on my right side even with painful stimulus. My leg hurt when I was walking. Charlotte took me to have my arm scanned and I was told that the problem was caused by a build- up of calcium in the shoulder joint. Physio was suggested and for the next 18 months this became an important part of my day. The exercises took one hour to carry out and I always did them, at least once, but if I wasn't otherwise busy up to three times a day. I now have minimal problems with my joints but have no idea whether my strenuous efforts have helped or whether things would have improved anyway.

I persuaded the rehabilitation unit to allow me home at weekends when the therapists weren't on duty. I only survived the whole thing because of this. I think it was my brain damage that made me feel like I did. The staff were great and

I don't remember witnessing anything that I was concerned about.

Antidepressants helped very slowly. For a time I felt they helped me cope but I still had underlying thoughts that I wish I had died and not had to put on an act in front of family and friends. I took the pills for over a year before I thought that the depression had improved. I was starting to feel I had a future. I am still not sure exactly what the future will bring and what I will end up doing with my life. However I now know that I have a future and no longer feel unhappy with who I am. It would be easy for me to leave out the account of my depression from the story, but it is part of what happened. Also if anyone reads this, and knows the pain of depression, this account may make them see that for me it came to a complete end eventually. I so hope it can happen to them.

At last I came to the end of my time in Sevenoaks. I was so pleased to be discharged but knew I would miss the staff. So home was good but as I have said, the depression continued for a time.

I was very worried about work. I knew I wasn't going to be well enough for some time and recognised that I would have to resign from my CEO post. I hated doing this and still feel sad about having to do it. It was the right thing to do at the time but as I have progressed it's become more difficult for me to come to terms with. It's hateful not being at work all day. It seems that everyone is at work so who do you spend time with? I could talk for ages about how difficult this has been for me but the end result is I hate it so much. However I volunteer for several organisations. I am doing very basic jobs at the moment but I have to build back up to what I am capable of achieving. Sadly, outside my volunteering roles, I have found discrimination against me as a head injury patient. There are people who make assumptions that I can't achieve certain things. I recognise that in some cases they may be right but in others they are wrong and the decisions about these things should be mine.

In the early days of being home again I was exploring the house and its contents and came across some of my belongings from the accident. For example I found my wedding ring and some other jewellery which had been taken off me after the accident and given to John. He had put them in my bedside cabinet and I had forgotten all about them, although I did remember them when I found them. One day I found a rather nice notebook and looking inside I realized it was a diary written by my children at my bedside when I was fully ventilated and unconscious. Reading what they wrote at that time has helped me a great deal as I had no awareness of that period at all. As well as highlighting for me what had happened it also gave me a deeper understanding of what my children had gone through and how they had coped. I have included the whole notebook as an appendix if you would like to read it – it is particularly interesting as it clearly shows their different personalities and ways of coping Clearly I have made an incredible recovery from my accident and can talk and mobilise fully. In fact if anyone met me for the first time and didn't know me they perhaps wouldn't realise what a dramatic experience I have had. However I am left with a few physical challenges which, despite my vast improvement, are becoming more noticeable as I progress and wish to move forward.

While in Sevenoaks I was told that my accident had caused a severe sight problem as I had lost one quarter of my visual field in both eyes. However in the early days I had not appreciated the significance of this. When I was discharged from hospital there were a few occasions when John saved me while crossing the road, by quickly pulling me away from oncoming traffic. Although they were near misses I didn't think it was my eyesight that was the problem.

It was at Josh's graduation celebration in Canterbury when I realised that my sight was a problem needing to be faced. I was walking fast across a pedestrian crossing when I walked straight into another lady who was on my right side. She was texting on her mobile and didn't see me. Although this was a small incident it made me realise that I simply couldn't see things at the right side of me. I researched it a bit and it seems that the brain makes up the bit it can't see. So if the road is clear in the ¾ area it can see, it makes a total picture of a clear road. This can be a problem if the car is in the blind spot. I had another accident at home when I fell over a piece of garden furniture which again was on my right side. This time the accident hurt.

I knew I wasn't blind but I wondered if Kent Association for the Blind might know a charity that could help me. I rang them for advice and was told by a lovely receptionist that they saw all people with sight challenges. A key worker came to see me and was fantastic. After fully assessing me she recommended a white cane. I felt I didn't really need a cane but we went for a walk with it to try it out. It's fantastic because it informs me if there is anything on my right side to avoid. It allows me to walk faster knowing that it's safe to do so. Obviously I had unconsciously been walking more slowly to protect myself from injury. People still say unhelpfully to me that when my confidence grows I can get rid of the stick, not realising that it's not used as a confidence aid but because I can't see a quarter of what I look at. I have had other help and advice from KAB and have recently applied to be a volunteer for them. If I can give back a little of what I have had I will be pleased.

My other difficulty has been a severe balance problem. I remember walking into Maidstone and finding the whole world was spinning around me such that I wasn't sure where the front really was. Looking back it was so scary. Eventually I was seen by a balance specialist and have been helped by valuable physio and the prescription of a special diet. It's a nightmare diet but I have stuck to it (even though a few friends have said they think it unnecessary) as I want to get as well as I can.

These are my physical disabilities but I have some cognitive challenges to cope with as well. What is it about my cognition that is the biggest problem for me and my family?

The difficulty is that it's hard for me to highlight what my challenges are as they are ever changing. Each month, sometimes each week, I realise I can do something that I wasn't able to do the last time I tried and thought about it. So I could write at length about the problems I have today, but by the time you read it they could have improved significantly. I think that's the hardest thing to come to terms with, that I don't know who I am anymore. Not sure what I am capable of, what I can do or achieve.

As I have said I refused the cognitive testing. I was aware that it wasn't normal not to know who the prime minister is. I didn't want reminding or need a test to prove what I couldn't do. I was deeply upset that I couldn't remember well or do everything I used to be able to do. I realised that the life I knew and the things I could achieve were now gone, maybe forever. I found it deeply upsetting when I received comments from people saying that I couldn't do something. Inside I felt the same person but suddenly I wasn't treated the same. People treated me differently in so many ways- one painful way was not valuing my opinion and thinking me wrong if my view simply differed from theirs. I wonder if it would have been easier if I had physical challenges like missing legs or arms. For me it was only my damaged brain which was the problem, which to look at you couldn't see. However I had lost the person I was. I am not saying that having huge physical difficulties is easy but losing the person one is, is also massively difficult and I feel not understood by many. People thought that as I had physically improved I should be thankful and realise how lucky I was and just get on with it. They did not understand that I had lost me. I feel Kate died in the accident and in time I am sure I will grow to like the replacement but I know that the old Kate has gone forever.

When I was in hospital I knew who the children were and also close family and friends. But I kept not being able to find the word I wanted and although this is gradually happening less and less often, it does sadly still occur. It's frustrating when I want to say it but the words won't come out, or I say it wrong. Hannah has highlighted in her account that I do this. For example I told John the other day that food was spilt in the washing machine and it needed cleaning. John asked why and I said the children must have boiled something over. Of course I meant the microwave. John was confused and I was frustrated that he didn't seem to understand what I was saying. We had a long heated discussion and then I realized that again it was my choice of words causing the misunderstanding. Of course we can all do this sort of thing occasionally. My problem is that it happens regularly.

My memory has improved but I still don't remember, for example, going to certain restaurants, whereas other restaurants I remember well. There doesn't seem to be a reason why one memory is intact but the other isn't.

I don't remember the accident itself but neither can I remember the four months of my life around it. People came to see me in hospital and I don't remember them coming at all. I remember previous significant things like the children being born but not everything in the past. I am hopeless at quizzes and games. We play a lot as a family. I never get the question right. I usually just don't know but if I am lucky I realise I do know but am much slower than everyone else. Again I find this a huge challenge. It would be easy not to play so my shortcomings are not noticed. However I like being with the family and playing games is a great way to be together. It would be easy to withdraw from all social situations as I hate standing out. However I push myself forward as I recognize deep down that it's not my fault. It could happen to anyone else and so I don't withdraw. I hope that I still have something to offer people even if it is rather different now. I know nothing about current affairs. I have little history of what is happening in the world to build on as my memory has been so affected. When people listen to the news they are building on what they already know about a subject. But what if you don't already know anything!? I have recently found an app which sends me ten news stories every morning and ten at night. I now ensure I read these every day to try to build my knowledge back up. As my memory is poor I have an app that sends me cognitive tests which I do every day. They take the best part of an hour to complete but I think I am very slowly improving. They give me results compared to other users. I used to score in the bottom 10 per cent but I now score at 65 per cent. I am slowly improving.

Face recognition is also a problem for me. If I knew someone well before the accident I would recognise them now. I may not remember their name but I know them and fully remember how we link together. However I really struggle to recognise new contacts. I may spend all day with someone one day and the next day, if we meet, it is as if I have met a stranger. For some reason it is worse for some people than it is for others. I need to have met a person about ten times before I recognise them in the future. I don't feel I could work because of this significant problem. I recognise people's jewellery, hair styles and tone of voice - it's just the face I can't remember. However I have become good at hiding this. I had a long conversation with someone at a station the other day and when we had parted I told my friend, who was with me, that I had no idea who they were. She couldn't believe I didn't 'know' the person. Often a conversation will give me clues as to how I know someone. This time it hadn't. They clearly knew me well! It has got me into trouble once. I met a man pushing a bike. As I know many cyclists I assumed I 'knew' him but couldn't recognize him. It was a long way into the conversation before I realised we didn't know each other. I was being chatted up, which I guess is a first time since the accident.

So my cognitive problems remain a challenge despite vast improvement. However I also know I am a very, very lucky woman. I have a family who have stuck by me and clearly care about me. Having spent a while highlighting the challenges I face, it's important to record that certain areas of my life have actually improved since my accident. I have always loved John but I feel closer to him now than I did before my accident. I realise how well he responded to the crisis we were in. He cared about me so much and he has encouraged me to move forward. He has achieved this by expecting me to return to as near normal as possible. For example, he bought me a tandem to race on and this fairly simple act has made all the difference as I can safely ride again. My eyesight would never allow me to ride my own bike but we have actually raced the tandem and now I am as physically fit as I was prior to the accident. We cycled to Bordeaux last summer and next summer we are cycling in the Alps.

I have also realised how well my children have turned out. From what I have been told they were amazing when I was ill. However I am most proud of them because although they showed signs of distress, when I might have died or remained unconscious, they also showed signs of being able to recover and get on with their lives. As a parent that is my job, to bring up children who can move forward in life without me. I am so proud of them all.

I bought my parents a local calendar for Christmas the first year. I was still unwell on the whole but I had an amazing idea. I wrote in the calendar that the present would be that we would go and visit the area where each picture was taken.

Each month we have a special day out and have been all round Kent. So the accident has enabled me to spend time with my parents. I used to be too busy but now I have time to spend with them in a fantastic way. I also have some new close friends. It's funny that some people have been amazingly supportive. Karen has supported me to write this account. She has also checked the grammar and spelling for me. Others have had their dinner break with me, for example, so I am not alone all day. (I was alone a lot in the early months). There are so many who should be proud of what they have done. Others have found it difficult and have left me alone to suffer or have simply not understood.

Since my accident I have found myself in a strange situation. Having spent the last thirty-five years supporting patients and families with health conditions (and hoping very much that I have done this as well as possible) the roles are now reversed. I have received support and care from a vast number of professionals, supporting my cognitive and motor challenges and my sight and balance difficulties. I see from a different perspective what good care looks like and what a difference it can make. I also have a better understanding now that different people need different help- I recognise that the real skill is finding out what each individual requires and providing that appropriately. I myself have been extremely lucky and have had superb care from a range of different professionals- physios, the Kent Association for the Blind rehabilitation worker, a balance doctor and physio, my GP and the practice in general……….. Thank you to you all.

Because my life has changed dramatically I have had to find new ways to move forward positively and achieve things of value. Over the last few months I've started to think about what I can achieve and what's important to me. Reassessing what is truly important in life has been a very valuable lesson. In my previous life I was intellectually able to perform at a very high level and lead a service for the whole community. I now find I am not able to do this and have often belittled what I have managed to achieve. Yet over the last few weeks I have come round to thinking that I can only be judged on what use I make of my abilities, not on how great my achievements are. Although I was very upset to have to leave work, the extra time I have gained has allowed me new opportunities and I am trying to enhance my life in as many ways as I can.

I have trained as a fitness instructor and now volunteer at a local gym. I am encouraging those with disabilities to engage in fitness. It gives me something else to think about and last week a school for children with special needs attended the gym and I undertook my first fitness class by myself. At the moment I don't feel well enough to work but I can offer something as a volunteer.

I have talked about the problems I have had to cope with since my accident but what has helped me in my recovery? Apart from people who have supported me so well, a couple of things have also made a big difference. I have valued volunteering. I love it as it enables me to be part of a team and reduces the social isolation which can be so damaging. Being a cyclist has helped me recover in so many ways. Firstly the improvements I have made physically have, I am sure, occurred because of the demanding physiotherapy that I have undertaken daily over the last 2 years. This has fitted into my training routine in the same way as my previous cycling training did. I used to spend time training and just carried it on. It meant that I continued to improve. Luckily it worked and, for example, my arm movement / function has improved to near normal. My balance has also improved, again, I am sure, because of regular exercise. But perhaps the greatest benefit that physical activity has given me is my improvement mentally. So the tandem has been really important. John and I race on it and have managed some good times, sometimes achieving at 25 mph over a 50 mile course. Such physical activity has helped my mood improve and there is evidence to suggest that physical activity helps with depression. I still sometimes have bad moments but overall I am learning to like the new Kate Bosley.

So cycling did almost kill me but without a doubt it has enabled me to survive. I love it!!

So where shall I end? The decision is a difficult one as all the time I am slowly gaining skills and continuing to improve - not back to how I was but back to a "me" I am proud of and like.

I used to be a normal woman who invested her time and passion in her family, cycling and her career. I then had a major event which challenged all of those areas of my life. I used to manage a home and four children, cycle and race my bike regularly and also work at a senior level for a charity. I was left with none of these available to me and each of them challenged.

With determination and hard work all the physio I did has paid off. Love and understanding has allowed me to be a useful wife and mother again. Sight prevents me from ever cycling solo again but does not stop me riding on a tandem! John and I have even raced on it and I feel like any other cyclist when we do. Volunteering has also allowed me to be useful in my own way - so slowly I am getting there and can now see a useful future for myself. So my message is, "Don't give up, always try! You'll never know what you can achieve unless you do!"

I went to see the new Cinderella film the other night. The film is based around a message which Cinderella is taught by her dying mother and which, despite a challenging life, she tries to live by. That message is 'Be courageous and be kind'.

It struck me as strange, as in my own way that's what I have tried to live by, especially since my accident. I have tried to be courageous and at times it has tested me enormously but its importance has always been with me. Kindness has always been central to what I aspire to.

I have witnessed so much kindness myself. Little things people have done for me now make such a difference. If you have showed kindness to me, and you may not even been aware that you have, thank you. Perhaps you moved out of my way when I was walking down the street with my white stick. Thank you.

I am still moving forward and therefore the end of the book doesn't really feel like it's the end of my saga. Having said that I could continue writing my updates forever and the bulk of what I have achieved has already happened. My key message is "aim to develop". The balance between accepting who I am now and continuing to move forward and improve has been a difficult one. So on one level it's important that I learn to accept that life is bound to be different when something like this happens. At the moment I am not capable of things I once found easy. However alongside this acceptance is the real need to continue to strive, grow and develop. I must never ever give up. I am still growing and developing, I am becoming a new me. Let's hope I can meet this challenge and allow it to make a difference!!

Be courageous, be kind!

POSTSCRIPT

September 2015

So the book was published on Kindle. I had some good reviews and I decided to get some feedback, make some changes and then get it printed. I got various comments but all had the same suggestion - Tell them what you have recently achieved, what you are now capable of! The trouble with responding to this is I may constantly have updates of things I have attempted or achieved as I have said before. Head injury recovery is very lengthy but 3years is the most commonly quoted length of time to gain the most recovery. As it is 2 1/2 years since my accident I'll include these recent updates:

We've had a fantastic summer. I bet you can guess. We spent it cycling!! Firstly we have a new Tandem - it's unique, purpose built and the best tandem money can buy! Its first trip was to Amsterdam We cycled from Kent, up to Harwich, took a ferry across to the Hook of Holland and then cycled to Amsterdam. Then we cycled home, via Calais. It was a good warm up because we planned a more difficult trip later on in the Summer. We cycled with Ant (Son-in-law), Hannah and her boyfriend Simon. Once completed we had a few days at home and then we set off to the Alps. John is going to tell you about the trip there which was an amazing event.

The Raid Alpine organised by Polka Dot Cycling - this was to be the biggest challenge since Kate's accident.

What is the Raid Alpine? A route designed by Georges Rossini that starts from Thonon-Les-Bain on Lake Leman (Geneva) runs over about 700km, over 30+ Cols (many used for the Tour de France) and finishes in Antibes on the Med. As an official Randonnee a medal is awarded to anyone who completes it.

Who are Polka Dot Cycling? They are an amazing cycling travel company (http://www.polkadotcycling.com) organising the Raid Alpine trip is just one of their amazing cycling holidays (quite a challenging one!)

Day 1 safely negotiated through rain and low clouds! Started with 3 Cols the Moises, Terramont and Jambaz that really blended into one long climb. Around the corner was the Col de Ramaz, climbing up gradients up to about 10%. We got very cold on the decent. Water in our shoes, etc. but we got down safely! That left just 2 climbs to go, the Col de la Croix Verte and finally up to Megeve in the sun! Wet, Cold and Kate had sore knees and some abrasions -but loved it!

Day 2 dry! Yippee

The day started with a run down to the bottom of the first climb, the Col de Saises . The group stayed together for the most part up the Col and we had some fast descending before a coffee break. It was then the Col de Pre. Not heard of it - it's an amazing and beautiful climb with lots of hairpins, through Alpine meadows and Chalets, but it's steep - Ave7.6%. After that you need a good rest- no chance, quick snack at the bus, a few KM around Lake Roseland then straight into the Cormet de Roseland - Rest time? Basically a delicious baguette eaten in about 5 mins before heading for 20km of very fast descending, about 10km along a Valley, then straight into a long 20km climb up to Val d'Isere. Very deceptive - does not look steep and you wonder why you are going so slow! Kate complained at one point that we were going downhill but only managing about 15kph - I pointed out that cyclists going in the opposite direction were managing to freewheel uphill!. Kate's knees have supports on to ease the pain but have started to cut into her skin - always has something to moan about!

Day 3 a bit of a challenge!

The day began with completing the remaining 15km of the Col d'Iseran. This actually went very smoothly and quite quickly, and on the ascent a Marmot ran across the road just ahead. (Marmots are large squirrels and live in mountainous areas, such as the Alps. Marmots typically live in burrows - Most marmots are highly social and use loud whistles to communicate with one another, especially when alarmed. marmots are usually found in groups of cyclists, there's always at least one!). This was followed by a long descent of about 15km and a coffee break before about 35km against a head wind to the foot of the Col de Telegraphe. Here we quickly ate some sandwiches, haribo and fluids to get us up the next two climbs! The Telegraphe was a great climb which we rode up steadily. Reaching the top after about 12km we quickly stocked up with more fluids and Haribo before a short 5km downhill led us to the monster 18km climb of the Galibier. The Telegraphe had been in the Sun, the clouds descended on the Galibier with about 5km to go. The temperature plummeted, and by the top we were already getting cold. Extra layers were quickly put on before the following 24km descent. The tandem was shaking as we shivered and it added extra challenge to a day that was about 156km long with three of the biggest climbs thrown in!

Day 4, I think. Polka Dot cycling (Stuart!) describes this as a recovery day. So that'll be only 100km then - and just two climbs. The first, the Col d'Izoard started almost straight away, only 19km to the top! Glorious sunshine, nice easy up - well, the first half anyway! Then the obligatory downhill and technical 8km section followed by a beautiful 30km or so through gorges to the foot of the Col de Vars. Beautiful day now very hot so plenty of fluids needed for another 19km climb and more stunning scenery. This only left the 8km technical followed by another 20km to Jausiers (which worryingly seems to be at the start of the Col de la Bonnette - the highest pass in Europe). Anyway, for now, a very nice stop in Le Chateux. Recovery? I guess so! In fact Kate just wore my leg warmer today and her knees have begun to settle down (of course her saddle is causing a few problems!)

Day 5

Jausiers to Valberg, over the highest pass in Europe, the 26km of the Bonnette de Restefond fantastic climb followed by 8km of decent (or was it 14?) Kate's given up screaming on the downhills! 30km along a Valley before the final climb, the Col de Cuillole. A few tired riders looking forward to an easy downhill day tomorrow - Tomorrow Antibes (near Nice)

Day 6 - Finished! Stage 6 of the Raid Alpine complete - we reached the Med! At what point we came to believe today would be easy! 156km from Valberg to Antibes we had thought would be downhill! No, we climbed the Col de St Raphael for 8km, the Cols of Castellaras, Sine and Ferrier for 17km, the Col de la Beine over 4 km and the Col de Pilon for 9.5km. It should then have been a straightforward 35km ride to the sea, but our gear cable broke and we were stuck in our top gear for the rest of the journey! Excellent trip though. We have cycled about 500 miles and over 17,000 metres of climbing .

Very well organised by Polka Dot - highly recommend them. The group dispersed on the final day - strangely emotional. People you'd never met before had completed a significant challenge with you and it's sad to say goodbye (though ongoing contact through Facebook or Strava is likely these days). A great bunch of people and that included the 'guides', who are the best travel agents and love cycling themselves. And 2 1/2 years after nearly dying, what an incredible achievement for Kate!

So that's what we have been up to. I hope it highlights that moving on from a head injury is possible. Polka dot cycling were with us when we were in the biggest challenge of our lives, how lovely it was to be with them when we achieved another type of challenge. One that we both enjoyed so much. So there is a life for us and challenges to enjoy and succeed at. In so many ways we have been lucky!

THE EMAIL STORY

(Geoff was Kate's Cycling coach)
On 20 February 2013 16:49, John Bosley wrote:
Hi
I'm in Tenerife. I'm afraid Kate has come off her bike on Monday and is in intensive care in hospital. It doesn't look good, Geoff. I think it only fair to let you know and I guess if you could let some key people know as my TT secretary duties are not going to happen. For now it would be best I think other than that to keep it confidential. Some family and friends do not know yet - it's hard to talk.
John
(TT stands for time trialling a type of cycling race which John was involved in organising locally.)

On Behalf Of Geoff W   **Sent:** 20 February 2013 18:24
To: John Bosley   **Subject:** Re: Kate
John
What can I do to help?
Do not worry about the TT duties. I will ensure that we quickly get a team together to take over from you.
Your priority is Kate.
Again, please let me know what I can do to help.
Geoff

(Cycling Friends)
From: Geoff H   **Sent:** 20 February 2013 19:51
To: johnbosley   **Subject:** Geoff W
Dear John

Geoff W has just given me the news of the dreadful accident. Our thoughts are with you, Kate and your family. Please do not think of anything to do with TT Sec. I will deal with anything that needs doing.

When you do have time I would be grateful of any update, if there is anything we can do please let us know.

Geoff and Carol

On 20.02.2013 22:43, John Bosley wrote:

This is just a quick contact to some of our closest friends. Kate has had a serious accident and is fully sedated in intensive care in a hospital in Tenerife. The accident was on Monday, a crash on her bike which resulted in a severe blow to the head. I'm afraid it is difficult to talk about this at the moment but I just wanted each of you to know. It looks likely to be weeks or even months to see if or how she recovers. Please be cautious. I have told Charlotte, Hannah and Josh but Sarah is away with school and they will see her and look after her when she returns on Saturday. I don't want her to find out by accident.

Love John

(John's father also called John)
On 21 Feb 2013, at 06:37, "John Bosley wrote:

Found message on answer phone from Bernard - I guess he got my number mixed up with yours.

Cheers, J/Dad

Sent: Thursday, February 21, 2013 8:58 AM **Subject:** Re: answer phone

He may have been contacting you about Kate, Dad. She is in intensive care in a hospital in Tenerife. It really doesn't look good. I have spoken with Josh, Charlotte and Hannah. Sarah though is away skiing with school and I don't want her finding out by accident. I want the kids to look after her when she gets back.

Love John

(Annie Kate's secretary)
From: John Bosley   **Sent:** 21 February 2013 08:26
To: Ann B   **Subject:** Kate
Hi Ann,

I'm sorry to contact you like this. Kate has had a serious accident that resulted in an impact to the head. She is fully sedated in intensive care in Santa Cruz, Tenerife. This happened on Monday - I wasn't with her. It doesn't look good Ann. I would appreciate it if you would inform the Chair of Trustees. At the moment I would appreciate confidentiality. I have spoken with my 3 eldest children but Sarah is on her ski trip. My preference is that the 'children' meet her on her return and look after her, they have the support of Kate's parents, but I don't want Sarah finding out by accident.

John Bosley

From: Ann B   **Sent:** 21 February 2013 09:22
To: John Bosley   **Subject:** RE: Kate
Dear John

I am so sorry. I have spoken to Roger (the chair) who sends his love and best wishes. We will keep this confidential until we hear further from you.

John, I don't really know what to say. I know it is trite but Kate is my friend so please do not hesitate to let me know if there is anything at all that I can do to help you or the family. I would really appreciate it if you could keep in touch when you can, but I don't want to add to your burden. My love and best wishes to you and Kate.

Annie

(John's father and his wife Nina)

From: John Bosley **Sent:** 21 February 2013 09:31

To: John Bosley   **Subject:** Re: answer phone

John, we are both thinking of Kate and all of you and please give her our love.

Love Dad and Nina

From: John Bosley   **Sent**: Thursday, February 21, 2013 9:40 AM

To: Bernard Wilson **Subject:** Thank you

Thanks for your text Bernard. This morning I have e-mailed Kate's work and mine. Yes, good idea to cancel Southwold. The kids have been brilliant, I'm so proud of them. I had spoken with them but was becoming incoherent so I did send them an email to describe my thoughts which they may have shared with you, but if not, this is what I wrote: "I think the Hospital is called Candelaria, it's the university hospital in Santa Cruz, Tenerife. It's a long way from the hotel so I am staying a bit closer in the house of the organisers. I am fine. It's difficult but they are looking after me. This next bit is hard to read but I will give you the facts as I see them. Mum is sedated and the doctors only speak a little English. But I can see that Mum is comfortable and out of pain though she is unconscious. They are sure that she has severe brain damage. They will occasionally, over the coming weeks, reduce the sedation to assess her. But this is going to take weeks, one even mentioned 6 months. What I am not sure is what this means for her in the long term. I don't know whether the damage is so bad that she may not survive or whether she may survive but have mobility problems, sight problems, mental impairment etc. I don't know and they don't know. It isn't very helpful I know. There are no other injuries to other organs or bones etc. I will tell you what I think about you coming out here but I am not telling you what to do so please just read my thoughts and still decide for yourselves. There are no rights or wrongs here. I don't think now is the right time to come. This is partly because I hoped you would be there for Sarah who is much younger than you all. But it is also the reality of the situation. Mum will not know that you are here. Visiting is only 7-8pm and it is intensive care so there is nowhere to sit and you can't get very close to Mum. But I understand that you would want to see her. I think that if things progress there will be times when Mum becomes semi-conscious. This would be good progress but might be weeks away. At that time I think she will need people. I don't expect that I will come home yet, but if Jan and Bern decide to come out then I would want to come home to be there with you all. That would mean that we could come out when Mum might need us, rather than for our need. I hope that makes sense."

That is what I said to them. I am also able to visit at 1pm each day just to receive updates from the Drs. Last night I did not visit as I knew that she was going for her third CT scan so I will get an update today. But I don't expect any change to her condition yet.

I would like you to come over Bernard but I don't think there is an immediate rush for this. However, if you need to come then please do. I think that I may have more information over the next few days so that we can make some planned and logical decisions about what is best. BUT I am sure there are no rights or wrongs about this so please also do what you and Janet think best. (For now I want to know that Sarah is supported when she returns and it sounds like the kids are dealing with this).

Thanks.

Love John

(Kate's Father Bernard. a number of e-mails from him and her Mum Janet labelled B&J)

From: Bernard **Sent:** 21 February 2013 10:34
To: John Bosley   **Subject:** Re: Thank you

Dear John,

I think putting all this in an email was the right thing to do. Not only was it easier for you than speaking one to one, but also it means that we don't have to think "what exactly did he say?"

Not that it makes it any easier to read and take it in though.

I have talked to the kids again after receiving your email and they are wanting to come out straight away unless we are planning to do so. Of course, we are ready to come, but we feel that perhaps the children should go first as they want to. I think that Hannah and Josh are planning to go immediately, with Charlotte waiting for Sarah and then following on Saturday. That is the impression I have, though of course it may be changed by any difficulties they have with transport and accommodation. I will ring them again and offer transport when I've finished this.

Then when they have to come back, Jan and I could come out for a week or two, giving you the opportunity to come home. I don't know what long term plans you will make, I don't suppose that you do either. We will just have to take things one step at a time.

Alan has come round to be with us, and he had a talk with Charlotte too. I'll get this off to you now, and if you let me have a landline phone number, I'll ring when you want to talk.

With our love,B&J

From: John Bosley **Sent:** Thursday, February 21, 2013 10:54 AM

To: Bernard **Subject:** Re: Thank you

Hi again, The landline number is....I know it's silly but I don't want to overuse that as they are just a couple trying to run the holiday, now looking after me at the same time etc. and of course they take their business calls on the line. The mobile phone is working well now as I've had a play and it actually rings! You might want to speak with Jen though, she has done a lot for us and visits Kate with me,

    Love John

    (Kate's brother Alan and wife Cheryl)
    Sent: 21 February 2013 11:37   **Subject:** Katherine
    Hi John

    Just a quick email to let you know that we are thinking of you all. If there's anything that we can help with, then please let us know. Alan is currently with Janet and Bernard and helping them out. Alan has also spoken briefly with Charlotte on the phone this morning to check if they need him to do anything for them; at the moment they seem to have things under control. We send you both our love.

    Lots of love Cheryl and Alanxx

    To: Hannah Bosley   On 21 Feb 2013, at 11:13, John Bosley wrote:

    Another pair of jeans, A few pairs of T shirts (Corner cupboard near door) 4 or 5 spare underwear (Socks in top drawer, briefs in middle drawer!) Some more anti-histamines (one of my bedside cupboards) My beard trimmer and Head and Shoulders shampoo! (under sink) Josh's passport and EHIc card is probably in the drawer in my desk? I think that's it.

    Love dad

    From: Hannah Bosley **Sent**: 21 February 2013 12:18
    To: John Bosley **Subject:** Re: Some things
    Ok all packed, we will leave for Sarah's soon xxx Love you xx

    From: Bernard **Sent:** 21 February 2013 12:24
    To: John Bosley   **Subject:** Re: Thank you
    Hi John,

I'm sure you'll know by now that the kids will be out with you tomorrow. I'm thinking that we might come a week later, but Charlotte says she could stay 3 weeks and we could come after that. So not sure yet. We have to avoid mid-March as Jan has an important eye-injection date which she mustn't miss.

Love Bernard

From: John Bosley **Sent**: Thursday, February 21, 2013 6:19 PM
To: Bernard **Subject:** Re: Thank you

Thank you Bernard. We'll see how things progress. I think this is going to be tough for the kids.

I have spoken with the Doctor today. He thinks that they will begin to get a clearer picture of how Kate's condition is likely to progress next week some time. I have been advised by the insurers that this hospital is a good place for her to be. It has a very good reputation.

Love John

(Chairman (at the time) of the Hospice)
From: Roger **Sent:** 21 February 2013 18:47
To: johnbosley **Subject:** Kate

Dear John, Annie called me this morning and told me your news about Kate. I cannot tell you just how devastated we are and our thoughts and prayers are with you at this extraordinarily difficult time.

I decided to call Bernard and Janet and spoke to them for some time, from the Hospice, where I have spent the afternoon. They have filled me in on some of the practical steps with the children and particularly the arrangements to tell Sarah on her return from skiing. Although it will bring its own issues, I am sure having the support of your family around you when they arrive will be a source of great comfort in the coming days.

I said to Bernard and Janet - and will repeat the same to you - if there is anything at all we can do to help you, please just ask. It's hard to think straight at a time like this but even if it was just helping on any insurance issue (about which I know a little more than most) or any practical things to do with home, or getting family to and from the airport, we would just be happy to help in whatever way we can.

John, I just wanted you to know we are thinking of you both and are praying for the most positive out turn from this awful accident. Ring me at any time.

Best wishes and send all our love to Kate.
Roger

From: Bernard **Sent:** 21 February 2013 19:39
To: John Bosley **Subject:** Re: Thank you
Dear John,

Thanks for this latest news. We are going to wait until the weekend to see how the kids are taking things, and then we will probably book a flight and accommodation for late next week. This may mean we duplicate with Charlotte (if she stays 3 weeks as she may), but if we don't come then it will have to be almost Easter as Janet can't fly for a week after having her eye injections.

We had a very nice phone-call today from Roger, the Chairman of the Hospice. He rang us as soon as he had heard. He says that the Hospice is totally shocked by the news. We are thinking of you and Kate all the time,

Love   Bernard & Janet

(Friend of the family)
From: alisonm   **Sent:** 21 February 2013 20:05
To: johnbosley **Subject:** Re: Kate
Hi John

Do let us know if there is anything at all that we can do. I was on the point of checking out flights to Tenerife but Mum is in hospital with a broken hip at the moment and I cannot leave her - I really wish I could be there. If you need us to be there with Sarah any weekend then just let us know - or if any of the kids need help with anything while you are there.

I know it will be difficult but do update us when you can. Take care and give Kathy our love and love to you too. Ali and Pete

From: John Bosley **To:** alisonm
Sent: Thu, 21 Feb 2013 20:40   **Subject:** Re: Kate
Thank you. They are taking control, Sarah's the one I'm worried about but Josh and Hannah are flying out tomorrow and Charlotte has arranged to fly out with Sarah on Sunday!

It's going to be very difficult for them Alison,
Love John

From: alisonm **Sent:** 21 February 2013 20:55
To: johnbosley   **Subject:** Re: Kate
It is going to be very difficult for you too - so you just shout if *you* need anything and/or anyone to talk to or any practical help that we can give. Is there anyone from the cycling place around for practical support?

What is the name of the hospital where she is?
Lots of love Ali

(Lisa and Jason, Friends)
From: kentranger **Sent:** 21 February 2013 18:47
To: John Bosley **Subject:** Re: Kate
John that's dreadful news you poor thing.

Not sure what we can do to help (I'll obviously pray) but please let us know if we can do anything, particularly in regards to Sarah.

Hope you're managing OK, stay in touch
Love Lisa and Jason xx

(Doff and Ken, John's Mum and Step father)
From: Ken R **Sent:** 22 February 2013 08:21
To: John Bosley **Subject:** your message
John, Just got your message. Mum is very upset. Hope all goes well. Please let us know if there is anything we can do. Take care and keep your spirits up   Ken

From: alisonm   **Sent:** 22 February 2013 10:45
To: johnbosley **Subject:** Kathy
Hi John

I am trying to think of practical things to do when I am this far away.

The number for the British Consulate in Tenerife is (from within Spain) .... They should be able to give some support if you need it.

Take care lots of love Ali

(Friend)
From: Marianna   **Sent**: 22 February 2013 18:44
To: johnbosley **Subject:** Kate
Dear John,

I was immensely sorry to hear of Kate's accident. My thoughts and prayers are with you and all your family at this most worrying time.

Yours very sincerely,
Marianna

From: Bernard   **Sent:** 22 February 2013 19:19
To: John Bosley **Subject:** Re: Thank you

Dear John

We have just had the encouraging news passed on by Charlotte about Katie's progress. We're so pleased to have something positive to hang on to. I know it's going to be a long road yet, but let's hope that this is the beginning.

It's good too that you have Josh and Hannah with you. We expect to fly out in a week's time or a little sooner.

all our love,

B&J

From: John Bosley **Sent:** Friday, February 22, 2013 8:29 PM

To: Bernard **Subject:** Re: Thank you

Yes, we've just got back to our broom cupboard! It was nice for Hannah and Josh as there has been nothing up until this. It may not mean anything in the long term but, as you say, very nice to have something to hang on to.

Love John

(Friends of family)

From: bev t **Sent:** 22 February 2013 23:00

To: John Bosley **Subject:** Re: Kate

Dear John,

Such shocking news. Our love to you and Kathy. Our thoughts will be with you all.

Love Bev and Karl. Xxx

(John's mother and stepfather)

From: Ken R **Sent:** 23 February 2013 11:15

To: John Bosley **Subject:** Kathy

John,

How are you doing? Sue phoned and told us Hannah and Josh arrived OK and have been to see Kathy. She said Kathy yawned, opened her eyes and then went back to sleep.

Surely that has got to be a good sign. Maybe because Hannah and Josh were there.

We feel useless, not able to concentrate on anything.

Thinking of you all constantly. Keep us up to date.

Lots of love and hugs.   Mum and Ken

(Friend)

From: Bernadette **Sent:** 23 February 2013 12:14

To: John Bosley **Subject:** Re: Kate

Dear John,

I'm shocked and stunned at this terrible news. I don't know what to say. Poor dear Kathy. I am constantly thinking of you and the kids and the desperate situation you find yourself in.

I will wait for further news and I really appreciate you taking the time to let me know.

Much love to all of you.   Bernadette

If there were something I could do then I would want to help.

From: Bernard   **Sent:** 23 February 2013 17:45

To: John Bosley   **Subject:** Re: Thank you

Hi John,

I have just booked our flights for FRIDAY March 1st. We will arrive at the South Airport at 15.15. No doubt we can make our way to Santa Cruz by bus.

Can you book us in to your hotel? That seems sensible. Jan will have to return by March 12th, I could stay on. We have only booked single flights.

Love from us both, B&J

From: John Bosley   **Sent:** Saturday, February 23, 2013 10:02 PM

To: Bernard **Subject:** Re: Thank you

That sounds great Bernard. Yes the bus is the 111 which goes every thirty mins. Hannah and Josh are due to fly back that day and need to check in around 6pm. They wondered whether to meet you at 4pm for a bite to eat at the airport? I'll check C and S's hotel when they arrive and see how it compares 4 u, they are about 100m apart! Very convenient for a tram to the hospital and in quite a nice shopping street. Shall I book a room for a week then you can extend?

I might fly home then on the Sat or Sun so I will have chance to show you around! (I'd need to find somewhere to stay!) Then I can sort a number of things out and may go to work for a couple of weeks (short days) possibly with a view to returning with Josh and/or Hannah later in March ... But probably thinking too much detail here!

I have put a message on Facebook today so that friends and relatives know. I've kept it simple.

Love John

From: Bernard **Sent:** 23 February 2013 22:20
To: John Bosley **Subject:** Re: Thank you

Are they flying from the same airport then? If so, then – yes it would be great to spend a little while with them. Yes, please book for a week and then I'll see whether to stay on.It seems a long time to wait before we can be with you. I've never known days seem so long! We're trying to find things to do to keep us occupied – all normal activities have been forgotten about. It must be so much better for you now that you've got the children with you.

I hope that you were able to crack Kathy's bank account code!

Thanks for making these arrangements for us,
Love from B&J

From: Bernadette **Sent:** 24 February 2013 09:07
To: John Bosley **Subject:** Re: Kate

Hi,

It's good to hear some positive news, although it is hard for us to imagine what actually happened and of the brain injury sustained but I don't want to burden you with questions at this time.

You have a difficult day ahead. Talking to Sarah will be very tough and I keep thinking of her.

Please tell Kathy that we are thinking of her all the time. I'd like her to know that she is special to me and I want her to get better.

Being so far away from home is a huge additional stress. I hope the hospital is looking after you both well.

I know I said that I didn't want to bother you with questions but I must ask after Janet and Bernard. I am thinking of them also.

Love Bernadette and Paul.

From: Ken R   **Sent:** 24 February 2013 19:21
To: John Bosley   **Subject:** re:Kathy
Hi,

Got your message OK - thanks. Like you said, there are more things to hang on to now and it all sounds encouraging.

We called Alberto in Madeira today and he sends his best wishes to you all. Eddison and Dorothy send their best wishes also.

On a practical point, how are you for cash? Don't be afraid to let us know if we might be able to help. We will try not to pester you too much but we feel inadequate.

Love Mum and Ken

(Kate's cycling coach and friend)
From: Geoff W   **Sent:** 24 February 2013 16:16
To: John Bosley   **Subject:** Re: Geoff W
Thank you John

My thoughts are with you and for a full recovery by Kate. I have a cousin, Ian B, who divides his time between the UK and Tenerife. He is currently on the island for the next 6 weeks. He has expressed a desire to help if he can, be it in a tangible way or just as a sympathetic fellow Brit.

His mobile phone no: I hope this helps. Please let me know if there is anything else I can do. Geoff

(Cycling friends)
From: Geoff H **Sent:** 24 February 2013 19:48
To: John Bosley   **Subject:** Re: Geoff W
Dear John

Thank you so much for the news. Carol and I are praying for a good outcome for you. In the meantime all our thoughts are with Kate, you and your family.

If there is anything we can do please do not hesitate to ask.

Geoff and Carol

On 24 Feb 2013, at 22:26, John Bosley wrote:
Hi Bernard,

No baggage for the kids, they hope it'll be delivered tomorrow. Unfortunately their hotel is not very nice. To be honest neither is ours but at least it's nicely located and has free wifi. We did wonder whether to look for an apartment?

We have seen an advert for one at about 350 euros a week with 2 bedrooms and a kitchen. Does that sound a good alternative? It could make eating a bit easier? It probably costs about the same as a hotel room?

John

To: Bernard **Subject:** Re: Thank you
Hi Bernard, I have another money problem now. We have a travelex cash card that we use for our holiday euros but Kate manages it. I've gone to get out cash today and it doesn't

recognise the pin! I may be able to reset it but now need Janet's middle name and birth date!

John

From: Bernard **Sent:** 25 February 2013 07:51
To: John Bosley **Subject:** Re: Thank you
Hi John,

As if you didn't have enough to worry about! What a mess – no baggage and no money!

Well, Janet's middle name is MARY and birth date is …..

We have a French bank account, and we left about €….. in it when we sold Lespinet, so there won't be a problem when we arrive. Can you manage until then?

Last May we stayed in a splendid hotel in Benidorm when we were doing our Spanish research. We paid only €50 a night for half board for the two of us. The meals were buffets, and we found that we didn't need to worry about eating elsewhere. I must say that I was hoping we could do something similar in Santa Cruz rather than having to worry about finding food every day. But Tenerife may be a different proposition to Benidorm!

I'll have a look on the internet and see what I can find. By all means have a look at apartments, but wifi is going to be an essential I would think.

I'll get back to you later.

Love to you all,

B&J

From: <u>John Bosley</u> **Sent:** Monday, February 25, 2013 8:26 AM

To: <u>Bernard</u> **Subject:** Re: Thank you

Thanks, no luck. They worked but then it wanted to know the make of car we had 5 years ago and the street number of Kate's work address! I was getting at least one wrong.

This hotel is about €50 a night but no food included. Charlotte's is €50 a night but only breakfast and no wifi. She did find an apartment online that appeared to include wifi but perhaps if you look first, thanks,

John

From: Bernard   **Sent:** 25 February 2013 08:27
To: John Bosley   **Subject:** Re: Thank you

Just looked at a few hotels. In every one, the feed-back was awful! Haven't found one that people were happy with.

Must go to doctor's now, Jan has problems with a hand that keeps losing feeling, and we both need some help coping with the situation. Don't want to arrive being a burden instead of a help!

Will be back later   B

From: John Bosley   **Sent:** Monday, February 25, 2013 10:25 AM
To: Bernard   **Subject:** Re: Thank you

Ok sounds good. Locked out of the account I'm afraid.

I wondered if Kate had booked travel to Southwold. Do you have any info. on that so I can try to get a refund?

The problem with hotels here is that Santa Cruz is not the tourist part of the island, good luck with looking.

At the mo it looks like Charlotte may stay out here for a further 2 weeks. Josh will come home but may return within a week for a further 2 weeks. I will go home and sort Sarah out etc and try to put in a couple of weeks work, short days, and then come out again. Certainly Sarah and I will then be out for the 2 week Easter hol which starts at the end of March.

John

On 25 Feb 2013, at 10:13, "Bernard" wrote:

Hi John,

I've just spoken to Annie, Kate's PA. As we guessed, there is no number for the work address. But she suggested that as the postcode is ...., you might try xxx?

Just got back from the doctor. Jan has some pills for her hand and neck, and we both have sedatives to help us. He says that Jan must come back to keep her eye appointment, we were wondering if she could give it a miss this time. So she will return on the 11th or 12th, but I'll stay on.

I'm going to look for accommodation now.

Love to all, Bernard

Sent: 25 February 2013 10:55
To: John Bosley   **Subject:** Re: Thank you

Hi John,

Kate booked on the same train as us for Southwold. She was coming from Cardiff I believe, and I'm sure that she got Annie to do it all for her. So probably all mixed up with the Hospice. However, by booking in advance and getting cheap fares, we have no refund opportunity and presumably she doesn't either. You could use your travel insurance, but it's probably not worth it as it was very cheap. More important to get a refund on the accommodation I should think.

How important is it to be very near the hospital? I found a possible hotel 15k away down the coast. On the 111 bus route I think. I'm assuming you can only visit for the one hour you mentioned.

One practical question. Is it warm? What sort of clothing are we going to need?

Love to all Bernard

On 25 Feb 2013, at 11:19, "Bernard" wrote:

Hi John,

This is the best I've been able to find in reasonable distance of Santa Cruz.

There are some adverse comments, but these seem to be youngsters seeking the high life.

I'd like to book half-board for a week, then stay on or move if necessary. Could you give me your opinion? Is it too far away? Would you and the others use it? Don't want to impose my choice on the rest of you!

Will wait for your advice. Bernard

From: John Bosley   **Sent:** Monday, February 25, 2013 12:47 PM

To: Bernard   **Subject:** Re: Catalonia Punta del Rey Expedia

I think you'd be lucky to find anything like that in Santa Cruz. It depends how you will get about and whether you want to be stuck in a holiday resort.

Where we are it's probably about 500m to the tram that goes to the hospital. The tram is very nice and seems quite cheap (the kids have a weekly pass that allows multiple use for €14) so whether there is a concessions ticket? There also seem to be museums, galleries, shops to visit so very convenient. We've also now located a supermarket but, of course, no way of cooking in the hotel. So that's where half board is useful.

Swings and roundabouts isn't it!

On 25 Feb 2013, at 13:57, "Bernard" wrote:

Hi John,

This is a difficult decision to make from this distance. I think that the most sensible thing for me to do would be to ask you to book us in for a couple of nights where you are. That will give us chance to take stock of the situation and look at the pros and cons of staying somewhere perhaps nicer but less conveniently placed. However, it seems that one can get a better deal when booking online. So if you like to give us the details of where you are (or where you expect to be) I could do the booking from here. I imagine that the apartment option would not be viable at present with 7 of us!?

Please let me know what you think about this, B&J

From: John Bosley **Sent:** Monday, February 25, 2013 3:07 PM
To: Bernard **Subject:** Re: Catalonia Punta del Rey Expedia

No problem. Our hotel is the Adonis Plaza, Santa Cruz (I think Charlotte may already have sent links previously?). The Adonis Capital is opposite and is part of the same chain. I haven't booked any accommodation yet so theoretically I am homeless on Friday, I'm waiting to see what days Hannah and Sarah will be going home.

John

On 25 Feb 2013, at 15:27, "Bernard" wrote:
OK! I've booked for ONE WEEK starting March 1st. Breakfast included but couldn't see a half-board option. I thought that Hannah and Josh were flying back that same day?

Hope the luggage is sorted. Bernard

From: John Bosley **Sent:** Monday, February 25, 2013 8:46 PM
To: Bernard **Subject:** Santa Cruz and Kate.
Ok, well, that'll allow you to find out about the place!

Josh and Charlotte were in two minds about staying on but I think they've realised that staying in a hotel actually can be quite expensive. So I expect Josh and Hannah to still go on Friday. I will then probably look into flying back with Charlotte and Sarah on Sunday, leaving is going to be hard though. The highlight of each day is when I visit Kate.

No further medical update re Kate. I am due a phone call tomorrow to go into detail about how things are progressing. She has calmed down a bit today and is more relaxed again, possibly back on sedation. Every time I visit things are just a little different. Today her eyes appeared to be moving under her lids and we felt that she was responding to our presence, but not consistently. She also seems to be breathing more of her own accord. Her stitches are healing well and her hair has started to grow (the kids think she suits short hair!). I do hope for a proper review tomorrow.

A lot of people have expressed concern and love for Kate. I am not communicating too much but the last couple of nights I have been up until midnight trying to catch up with people. I'll leave off a bit now as it's a bit tiring. Let alone the emotional side of things with the children etc!

Bye for now,
Love John

From Bernard   **Sent:** 25 February 2013 21:21
To: John Bosley   **Subject:** Re: Santa Cruz and Kate.
Dear John,

We do appreciate your emails. Often, when we are asked about things, we refer back to something you have written a day or two before. So it's better really than talking in some ways.

Now, about the hotel. I felt that we should have somewhere booked, but had in mind your reservations about the place, and also about somewhere more distant. I've spent ages today combing the internet for somewhere better suited! However, this booking can be cancelled without penalty, so if you think that would be sensible, please tell me and I'll take action at once.

So it looks as if we will be sending you the news by next week. You certainly deserve a rest, though it can be very tiring back here just wondering what is happening to our daughter. I'm sure you realise that we are totally devastated by what has happened, so when we say that we understand what you are going through, you know that we really do.

We are getting enquiries from friends and relatives asking for the "latest news", and it's hard to have to say "no change as far as we know". I know it must be the same for you.

We have had another very kind call from Roger, and yesterday Lady M rang us. People think so much of Kate and are so concerned about all of us as a family.

So do you think that they removed the sedation yesterday? I got the impression somehow that she was in an induced coma and would be for some time.

I'm wondering whether not being enthusiastic about an apartment has made it difficult for Charlotte to stay on. If we rented an apartment, would she consider staying? I will ring her tonight and talk to her about it.

I'll let you go now!

All our love to all of you,

Bernard and Janet

From: John Bosley   **Sent:** 26 February 2013 16:07
To: John Bosley   **Subject:** Me again!

Just to ask how you all are - especially Kate, of course. Everybody is thinking of you.

Dad and Nina x

(John's eldest sister)
From: Sue Bosley   **Sent:** 26 February 2013 19:05
To: johnbosley   **Subject:** Hello

Hi John

Just spoke to dad so had a potted update.   Rob's parents & sisters send their love & well wishes & will want me to have told you that they are thinking of you all.

Kate's fitness and strength both physically & emotionally will surely give her the best chance on her road to recovery & she has everyone that knows her rooting for her.

Hope you & the kids are all holding up ok....we are here for anything you might need....however big, small or off the wall....just ask.

Love to you all from everyone here
Sue Xxx

From: Ken R   **Sent:** 26 February 2013 17:29
To: John Bosley   **Subject:** How is everything?

Hi, How is everything and in particular, is there any change in Kathy's condition? Have the doctors given you any further ideas?

I am sure most of the kids are coping well but how is Sarah in particular? As you suggested, it must have been a bit of a shock for her but at least she has the rest of her family around her.

I had a very friendly and caring message from Annie B at the hospice. Sent her one back but it looks as though they are doing everything they can to help.

We have realised that we do not know where you are on the island. No reason why we should of course but it is no good us looking at Google maps if we have no idea which town you might be in.

How long are the kids hoping to stay in Tenerife?

Finally, again, let us know if there is anything we might be able to help with.

Lots of love, Mum and Ken

From: John Bosley   **Sent:** Tuesday, February 26, 2013 9:56 PM
To: Bernard   **Subject:** Re: apartment ... nicky k?

I've been in touch with Nicky K. Do you know her? Kate's Doctor friend. She is on Tenerife with her husband for 10 days from Monday and would like to visit?

John

(Friends)
From: John Bosley **Date:** 26 February 2013 22:07:51 WET
To: Nicky & Phil K   Subject: Kate
The hospital (Candelaria), is to the right of the purple pin. Parking is horrendous but I found that if you turn right immediately at the point under the pin then there is plenty of parking around the little one way system. It's then about 100m walk to the entrance to the hospital (you actually enter through a gate at the back and follow the road around to the front of the building and the entrance which faces the sea). John!

From: Bernard   **Sent:** 26 February 2013 22:09
To: John Bosley   **Subject:** Re: apartment ... nicky k?
I think I may have met her once, I believe Kathy brought her orienteering some years back. I certainly know of her, isn't she from S.Africa? Yes, it would be good to meet up. Can you fix it?

The apartments that I found and sent to you are all taken.   Bernard

From: Bernard   **Sent:** 27 February 2013 14:26
To: John Bosley   **Subject:** Travel
Hi John, I've booked Janet's return for 12th March, Easyjet from Tenerife South at 12.05. Roger says that he will arrange for her to be met at Gatwick. That's a load off my mind!

I'll stay on until you return, which I suppose will be about the last week in March? When I know definitely I'll book my return too.

After we've had coffee with Josh and Hannah at the airport on Friday we'll take the bus to Santa Cruz. Will you be able to meet us at the bus station?

Nothing else to report from this end. Hope to hear how things were today in due course.

Love from B&J

From: John Bosley   **Sent:** Wednesday, February 27, 2013 4:30 PM

To: Bernard Wilson   **Subject:** Kate updates, Wednesday

Hi Janet and Bernard,

Some updates about Kate. I have spoken with the insurers' medical team a few times today. They have approved the tracheostomy as a positive way forward and they have confirmed what I have been told by the medical staff at the hospital. But they have also said that just because Kate is in a coma does not mean she cannot make very good progress and it will take time. They think that the tracheostomy will help to further stabilise her condition and allow them to assess when she can be flown home. They are pushing for this sooner than later and even talked of an air ambulance. So we could see her flying home with Janet or soon after ... That would be a positive step for all of us. So for now don't be booking up accommodation without options to cancel!

On 27 Feb 2013, at 17:10, "Bernard" wrote:

That's very encouraging news! We must have a good chat about what we should do about accommodation after our stay at the hotel runs out, and how best to maintain contact when you are gone. Thank you for keeping us in touch.

Love B&J

On 27 Feb 2013, at 20:43, John Bosley wrote:

We visited Kate this evening and it would be easy to say, 'same story'.

Having said that the children seemed very encouraged by the visit and feel that she shows little signs of responding to our presence. If we are looking for small signs of progress then, yet again, she made very small but new movements. Moving her left arm towards the centre of her body, moving her lip and also her legs occasionally. I know this is difficult to take in but the children love to see her and talk to her. We only go in two at a time but they talk to her as though she can hear us.

They hope to do the tracheostomy tomorrow and my insurers' medical team will attempt to call them on Friday for an update.

See you soon,

Love John

PS I have made sure they have the correct records and have given you as the local contact from Sunday. I have also said that we are based at the Adonis Plaza so, should you move into anything new just advise them.

Sent: 27 February 2013 22:06

To: John Bosley **Subject:** Re: Kate updates, Wednesday

Thanks John! Again, this is encouraging. It's so good to have these updates.

See you soon!

B&J

From: RS   **Sent:** 27 February 2013 **To:** johnbosley **Cc:** RK **Subject:** Sarah Bosley 11R

Dear Mr Bosley,

I am sorry to hear your news and I hope the situation improves, please keep us updated and we'll do what we can to help.

As requested, below is a table of work* that Sarah's teachers have emailed. There is also SAM learning and My Maths which is available online if Sarah would like to keep occupied.

With regards,
(Head of Year 11, Valley Park School)
Mr. R. Smith
* not included in this account

From: RSmith **Sent:** 27 February 2013
To: johnbosley **Cc:** RKirby **Subject:** Sarah Bosley 11R

Dear Mr. Bosley,

This is the second of two emails. Attached* is the relevant work that the teachers emailed.

With regards,
Mr R. Smith (Head of year 11, Valley Park School)
* not included in this account

From: Ken R **Sent:** 28 February 2013 15:43 **To:**John Bosley

Hi,

Thanks for all the information. Note you arrive home late Sunday. Will you be at school Monday? Have a safe journey home. Will speak to you on your return.

Give our best wishes to Bernard and Janet and apologise because we don't have their address or telephone number and could not contact them.

Let us know if there is any change but we will not contact you again until you get home.

Lots of love to all, Mum and Ken

(Cycling Friend)

From: Colin S **Sent:** 28 February 2013 16:11 **To:** johnbosley

John

Just heard the horrible news re: Kate. Our thoughts are with you all, if there is anything at all Sarah & I can do...you know we will.

C

Subject: Re:Kate **From**:jbosley **Date:** 28 Feb 2013 21:30:21 **To:** colins

Thanks for the message Colin. I don't think you are on Facebook are you? I'm using that to give occasional updates to friends and relatives. Kate is still in intensive care and has been unconscious for two weeks now. It seems cruel. She has no injuries below the neck at all and just some cuts to the face that have healed. Unfortunately the impact seems to have caused the damage. It's going to be long and slow to see if she comes out of this.

John

From: Col S **Sent:** 01 March 2013 08:34 **To:** jbosley **Subject:** RE: Kate

Hi John

We've got everything crossed and are thinking of both you and the family, we can't begin to imagine the pain you are all going through. I'm too old and grumpy to be on Facebook, I'll see if I can get one of the girls to add you or whatever it is you do, failing that it is good old fashioned email I'm afraid. As I said below we are local and if there is anything that needs doing this end, if we can help we will, please don't be afraid to ask.

Colin & Sarah

On 1 Mar 2013, at 07:38, Nicola K wrote:

Hi John

Thanks for the map. Any update or are things stable?

I'm heading back to Maidstone after work today then family to see over weekend then we fly Monday morning. Did you say you fly back Sunday?

Where have you all been staying? Have the cycle tour people been good? Was anyone else hurt? Did she get hit by a vehicle or some other accident? We'll contact Kate's Dad once we are settled in and see when it would be good to visit.

Thinking of you all love Nicky

On Mar 1, 2013 9:17 AM, "John Bosley" wrote:

To our knowledge there was no one else or a vehicle involved but unfortunately what happened wasn't seen. Kate's condition is stable. She has had a tracheostomy fitted to help maintain this and the insurers are beginning to look at potential for repatriation which would certainly be helpful for the kids who are running out of money! The tour company have been excellent. They put me up in their own house and took me back and forth to the hospital for the first half of last week.

Hannah and Josh fly back today and Janet and Bernard arrive. The rest of us fly back early on Sunday. We have been staying in two hotels in the City Plaza (hotel Adonis Plaza is the one I am in). Not great but excellent free wifi! Locally there are restaurants, shops etc and it's actually quite nice considering it's not really the tourist part of Tenerife.   John

From: Nicky K   **Sent:** 01 March 2013 09:22
To: John Bosley   **Subject:** Re: Kate

Oh John what a nightmare for you all. I'm glad people have been so helpful. Have a safe trip home. Hopefully you'll get Kate home soon too. 5hr flight's a bit too much for ease of visiting.

Kate was so wonderful visiting me I am thankful things have worked in such a way that I can get to see her.

Take care Nicky x

(Kate's father contacted the wrong John)
From: John Bosley   **Sent:** 01 March 2013 16:00
To: johnbosley   **Subject:** Bernard
Just had call from Bernard at airport who thought he was ringing you (again!). Thought I should let your know about it - he is very confused about things and could not speak because he was queuing for customs.

He has the wrong number but did not stay on long enough for me to help him.

Cheers Dad. X

 (TIME TRIAL Friend)
On 2 Mar 2013, at 08:51, Paul H wrote:
Hi John.

I heard the bad news last night about Kate. How is she doing?

Paul

From: J Bosley **To:** Paul H   **Sent:** Sat 2 March 2013, 9:12 **Subject:** Re: Kate
Hi,

She opened her eyes yesterday. First time in about 12 days. She also squeezed my hand when I asked her to. This is in contrast to lying in a coma so it's a start!

Thanks   John Sent from my iPhone

(Kate's secretary)
From: JBosley **Sent:** 02 March 2013 09:39 **To:** Ann B **Subject:** Kate update
Hi Annie,

We have some positive news at last, though early days of course. I took Hannah and Josh to pay their last visit before they flew home and when we walked in Kate had her eyes open! They weren't properly focusing but she was able to squeeze my hand on request. This is such a change and although it's very exciting it is only a tentative step. I imagine it may now be harder for Kate as she begins to realise her predicament. It made it a lot harder for Hannah and Josh to leave and likewise myself and Charlotte and Sarah only have today now.

On 2 Mar 2013, at 20:45, John Bosley wrote:
Hi, (Hannah and Josh)
Nothing to report really. Mum was asleep for both visits. We spoke to the Doctor again and he repeated that he was pleased and that she had slept for most of the day but had still woken for a while and squeezed his hand on request. She should start Physio on her right side tomorrow and may move onto a ward soon. Sounds like good news with the car, thanks. See you soon. I will drop off Charlotte at home and Ant is making us a meal so should be home by about 8pm I guess (don't block the garage!)
Love Dad

From: Hannah Bosley   **Sent:** 02 March 2013 21:47
To: John Bosley   **Subject:** Re: Mum
Thanks for the update, dad, that is very helpful. Xxx
  Saw your dad and Nina today. They both sent their regards and were very helpful.
Sue has asked that we pop by hers on the way home, so we will be popping in for a biccy and a cuppa.
See you soon, Miss you lots xx Hannah

(Cycling friends)
From: Pat H   **Sent:** 02 March 2013 21:25
To: John Bosley   **Subject:** Kate
Hi John,

Geoff has been keeping me in touch re your Facebook news about dear Kate. Ted and I send you all our best wishes and hope that you will soon have better news. One thing is that we bikies are tough cookies.

You are all in our thoughts and prayers,
Pat and Ted

(Lise is a friend but also the editor of the Milestone our cycling clubs magazine)
From: Lise T-V   **Sent:** 02 March 2013 22:49
To: John BOSLEY **Subject:** Kate in the Milestone?
Dear John,
I have been thinking of this for days. Since Kate is such a dedicated member of our club and has been in everybody's thoughts, hearts and prayers lately, I am thinking of dedicating this coming Milestone issue to Kate ... Kinda like one big get-well card.

I just want to ask you first and also if you would like to write a little bit about what happened and how she is doing now (up until a few days before print) as little or as much as you like ... and then I will ask everybody else to write their dedication and get well wishes to her. I would also fill the page with lovely photos of her.

We are many who just wish we could do more for Kate and if this in just a small way can be encouraging to her, it would be worth it. Hopefully it will be something she will be able to look back at as something positive in a difficult time.

Please feel free to say no if you don't think it is a good idea - it is entirely up to you.

With all my heart,   Lise x

(Kate's secretary)
From: Ann B **Sent:** 03 March 2013 20:11
To: John Bosley **Subject:** RE: Kate update

Oh John - my internet has been playing up. Just got your message. What good news. I know it is only tentative but still positive! She has such a will (sometimes wilful!) this must help her.

Thank you so much for keeping me updated. I really appreciate it. Much love to Kate and to you all. Call me if you need anything.

Annie x

From: JBosley **Sent:** 04 March 2013 08:28 **To:** RSmith
Subject: RE: Sarah Bosley 11R
Hi,

Just to confirm that Sarah is returning to school today. Her Mum is still in intensive care in Tenerife though may be moved onto a ward shortly. She is no longer in a life threatening situation however she may have significant injuries that cause long term disabilities, only time will tell. I give this information only in as far as it may be helpful that staff will understand if Sarah is emotional etc. I may travel back to Tenerife in a couple of weeks but her 21 year old brother is at home with her and older sisters are not far away.

John Bosley

From: RSmith **Sent:** 04 March 2013 15:32
To: John Bosley **Subject:** RE: Sarah Bosley 11R
Dear Mr Bosley,

Thank you for keeping us up to date. We have informed Sarah's teachers of the situation and we will keep an eye on her in the coming weeks.

Please email me if there is any further information.
Thank you, R. Smith

From: Lise T-V **Sent:** 04 March 2013 10:57
To: Undisclosed Recipients SFA

Subject: Get Well Wishes for Kate Bosley in the Milestone

Dear San Fairy Ann Members

You may have heard that Kate Bosley has had a serious accident whilst cycling in Tenerife. It has left her in intensive care where she has been unconscious for about two weeks. John has kindly informed us that Kate has now opened her eyes and shown signs of movement which is encouraging but limited.

Since Kate is such a dedicated member of our club and has been in everybody's thoughts, hearts and prayers lately, I have with John's permission decided to dedicate the next issue of The Milestone to Kate ...

John will write a little bit about what happened and how she is doing now and I kindly ask friends and colleagues to write your dedication and get well wishes to her. I will also fill the page with lovely photos of her.

We are many who just wish we could do more for Kate and if this in just a small way can be encouraging to her, it would be worth it. Hopefully it will be something she will be able to look back at as something positive in a difficult time.

So please, send me your contribution. Deadline is 11th March. Any nice photos you may have of Kate are very welcome too.

Kind regards, Lise T-V Editor of The Milestone www.......com

(Chairman of the Hospice)

On 4 Mar 2013, at 11:20, "roger@.......co.uk" wrote:

Dear John,

I trust the journey home for you and the "children" went well. I am sure it must have been tough to leave Kate behind - but then what truly fantastic news yesterday from Bernard! I cannot describe how uplifted I felt when reading his email. I'm sure there is a long way to go, but Kate seems to have begun to fight back as we all prayed she could. All the trustees have asked me to send you their continuing best wishes. I'm sure you have a thousand things to do, but it would be great to catch up with you if and when you have a minute. Any idea when it would be best to call?

Kind regards, Roger

On 4 Mar 2013, at 11:25, John Bosley wrote:

Hi Roger, we are very excited about this but it's within the context of where she was rather than where she may get to ... I'll explain myself when we speak. Any evenings should be OK to call. Perhaps not this evening as there is a lot of catching up to do. Thanks for all your support.

John

PS compared to Bernard I'm a bit of a spin Doctor so I am keen that people do not misinterpret her progress.

From: roger@.......co.uk **Sent:** 04 March 2013 12:02
To: John Bosley **Subject:** Re: Kate

Hi John,

Completely understand your caution. Indeed in sending it on to the Trustees last evening I quoted Churchill after El Alamein (it's not the end but perhaps the end of the beginning etc).

There's a huge hunger for information amongst all Kate's colleagues and we are just keen to make sure we feed that hunger with facts and not speculation.

I will give you a call tomorrow evening and in the meantime we will continue to keep everything crossed for further signs of progress along the long road to recovery.

Best wishes   Roger

(Cycling friend)
From: Dean & Sue   **Sent:** 04 March 2013 13:55 **To:** jbosley **Subject:** Kate

Hi John.

Desperately upset to have heard the news of Kate's fall/crash.

If I can do anything to assist you, Kate or your family please do not hesitate to contact me. I wish her a speedy recovery, and hope to see you all fit and well soon.

My thoughts go out to both of you. Please do not feel you have to reply.

Regards Dean C

If you need me ring !! Home ....Mobile ....Work ....

From: Bernard **Sent:** 04 Mar 2013 14:57 **To:** J Bosley **Subject:** Mon1pm

Dear John,

When we arrived we found Kathy wide awake and with her eyes clear and bright (no specs). At once a male nurse appeared and pointed to her lunch in bowls and pots. "She won't open her mouth" he said, "Please will you try to feed her!"

So Janet took up the spoon and a small pot of yoghurt and managed to get about three quarters of the pot down her. She didn't seem particularly keen to eat but we did our best!

We got some lovely smiles and strong squeezes, but I failed to operate my squeeze code system, she really isn't ready for that yet.

I talked to her a lot, explained where you all were and how you had been with her for nearly two weeks, and she seemed to understand.

Another doctor came (the third I have met) and said that they had done all that they needed to do in IC, and that she would almost certainly be moved to a ward today for rehabilitation. He reiterated that there was nothing wrong with any organs except the brain, and that they would be working to restore as much brain function as they could in her new ward. The male nurse told us to come tonight to the usual modulo and his colleague would tell us where to find her.

I don't think there's any more to add, except that conditions here are terrible. If we hadn't been hanging on to the railings coming up from the hospital we would have been literally blown away. I have never known such winds. There are men all over the city with long poles hacking down dangerous tree branches which haven't already fallen.

I imagine that you will pass this on to the kids. I'll write a briefer version for other friends and relatives.

So continued good news,

Love from us both,   J&B

On 4 Mar 2013, at 20:48, "Bernard" wrote:

Dear John,

Tonight they didn't let us in until nearly 6:30 and of course when we got to Modulo 1 we found as we expected that Kathy had been moved.

A very kind nurse took us to her new room through metres of corridors and up in lifts. I guess it was not the usual way visitors are supposed to go.

She is in room 844 in the main building, very high up and overlooking the pedestrian crossing we use. It is a room big enough for at least 2 beds, maybe 3, but she is on her own. It was very dimly lit, perhaps there is a reason for that. She is being fed by a tube in her nose, has an oxygen tube around her chin, and has a BP monitor on her finger. She managed a weak smile when we arrived, but was very sleepy and not ready for much interaction. Squeezes were not on the menu.

Everything is very different here. We can see a doctor each weekday at 12 noon, and visiting is anytime between 3.00pm and 9.00pm! The nurse said that we could feed her at mealtimes, though they would feed her if we weren't there. So we feel as though we are expected to be around most of the time! We'll be there tomorrow at noon and try to find out what the future is likely to hold. When will she be likely to be brought home, for example.

When we left, we had to ask to be shown the way out, and having managed that, we then went back in again to ensure that we had got it right! We end up coming down the stairs just past the cafe by that little lift.

How are we? Well, we have our ups and downs. Of course it's good news that Kathy is out of intensive care and we can't expect miracles, well not at once. But we were a bit depressed tonight to get so little response from her, and we were anxious at the way she sometimes struggles with the liquid which seems to collect in the tracheostomy apparatus, making her gasp for air. We fetched a nurse who seemed to think there was nothing to be concerned about. It should be removed in a few days. I suppose that we do miss you and the girls, the company and the chatter.

I have put together a contact group of friends and relatives to whom I will send an email once a day. It will be much briefer than this. Do you want me to include Annie and Roger in that group, or will you contact them after reading my email to you? And will you be sharing this with the children, or would you like me to include them in your daily email?

That's about it for today, I'll be back after we see the doctor tomorrow.

Love from us both,

B&J x x x

PS Got your text about phone problems!

From: John Bosley **Sent:** Monday, March 04, 2013 9:38 PM

To: Bernard **Subject:** Re: Monday evening

Thanks Bernard. It's a big step to move out of IC, didn't look likely just a few days ago! There should be fluid in the tube, I explained this to Janet. Is it more than that? It prevents the oxygen from drying out her lungs. And of course this isn't being pumped into her, she is breathing from it, unaided so sounds fine to me.

I am happy to keep Annie/Roger updated. I have asked Roger to call me tomorrow evening and I emailed Annie last night. And I copy/update the kids of course. I'm keeping things simple on Facebook because if you say she's out of IC or she's 'stable' then some people think that's it, she's fine now we can forget about her. I don't want that for Kate or for the kids. If this slow learning process takes months then it won't be nice if people don't realise how hard it all is, if they don't truly understand the reality of the situation.

I hadn't realised until the weekend that you weren't looking at my Facebook accounts. Every time I make a post, along with a picture, friends and relatives add some lovely comments, so if you get chance have a look back on them. They'll be nice for Kate to see one day.

It may be nice to visit Kate in the afternoon, perhaps she won't be so tired. I guess the longer visiting times will give you some flexibility about when to visit. If we had foreseen this I wouldn't have come home and I don't think Charlotte would. In fact she mentioned earlier that she'd love to come back out. Let's hope they fly her home soon.

Love John

From: Bernard   **Sent:** 05 March 2013 07:29
To: John Bosley   **Subject:** Re: Monday evening
Hi John,

Just a quickie to reassure you that we will be doing all we can to help Kathy. There is a sort of waiting room associated with all the rooms where the patients are. It's big and cheerful with large windows and a good view. I think that we will take our kindles and one of us will be with Kathy while the other is in the waiting room. That way we can keep up a relay of attention. There's a chair for one to sit by Kathy's bed. We will try the music today. I think she is tired in the evenings from the rehab which they have started in the mornings, so more time in the afternoon may be a wise move.

I've found and read the Facebook postings. Yes that is very encouraging to know all those people are thinking of us.

Jan wants you to know that the nurses were pleased with the way Kathy responded to Janet feeding her, and when possible she will continue to help in this way.

Love B&J

(Cycling friends)
From: Rosemary T   **Sent:** 05 March 2013 15:10
To: John Bosley   **Subject:** Re Kate
Hello John - just want to let you know we are both thinking of you and Kate, and, of course, your children and family. We have only recently heard about Kate's cycling accident.

If there's anything we can do which might help by way of support, please don't hesitate to contact us.

Kate is very much in our prayers.

Best wishes. Rose and Adrian T

(Kate's South African friend who lives in S A)

From: Joan L   **Sent:** 05 March 2013 18:52
To: John Bosley   **Subject:** Re: Kate
John-

I am so shocked and saddened to hear of Kate's accident. Thank you for letting me know.

My thoughts are with you and your kids at this terrible time and I only hope that soon she will show an improvement.

I will keep in touch with Facebook.

With thoughts and love   Joan L

From: Bernard **Sent:** 05 March 2013 20:11
To: John Bosley **Subject:** Tuesday update
Dear John,

Quite a day, and a good one at that!

We went to see the doctor at 12 noon as instructed. We were asked to wait in the waiting room which is very comfortable. We waited until 1.00pm when I was about to ask if we had been forgotten, when he appeared and took us into a consulting room. He had an A4 sheet report in front of him. I saw Kate's name spelled wrongly and put that right!

We had a long talk. He couldn't tell us much new, it was mostly me asking questions about how we can help best.

He said that she should be able to go to London next week if everything continued as at present. He was waiting for the agent to make contact again.

He reconfirmed that there were no complications apart from the brain damage. This, he said, was in both the frontal lobe and the parietal area. He couldn't say how much cognitive damage there might be, but there are as you know problems with feeling on the right side of the body. (However, when we saw her she was lifting her right leg right up).

On our way back to the hotel we had the phone call from Sarah, the agent who confirmed what the doctor had said about repatriation.

We went back to the hospital about 4.00pm and spent three hours with Kathy. As soon as we walked in we realised that there was a great improvement. Her eyes were wide open and clear and she smiled a big smile when she saw us. I got out her phone to play the music and she grabbed the phone from my hands and flicked the cover open! She enjoyed the music I'm sure, and I showed her the pictures we had brought. Sometimes her face seemed to suggest some puzzlement or confusion and her lips moved wordlessly. I was desperate to understand what she wanted to say. I tried the 1 squeeze yes, 2 squeeze no idea, but she didn't seem to respond. As she can control her left hand and fingers, I'm going to try an alphabet board tomorrow. Production work for Janet!

She still has the tracheostomy but there is no tube attached now. She has no attachments at all apart from the pulse rate monitor on her finger. Later on, a nurse came and connected some paracetamol drip to her cannula for half an hour or so. She was fed while we were there, though she didn't enjoy it much. I'm not surprised, it didn't look very appetising!

Her room is excellent. She has TV (we turned it off while we were there) and an en-suite toilet, shower and wash basin. This is obviously a new part of the hospital. There are no wards, just rooms of 1 or 2 people.

I can't overstate how much improved Kathy is. But as I say, I'm not sure how much she understands about her plight, where she is and why etc. I hope that this will get sorted out as she asks questions tomorrow. I don't want to give her information that she is not ready to receive, but I do want to answer the questions she clearly wants to ask.

Thanks for your texts. Roger had all the flight info for Janet and has presumably passed it on to Annie.

That's it for now,

Love from us both, B&J

(Cycling friend)

From: John Bosley   **Subject:** TT documents

To: "'richard n'"   **Cc:** "'Bill B'" **Date:** Tuesday, 5 March, 2013, 18:05

Dick,

I did submit police notices for the Club evening events this year (and   novice) to the police along with copies to the district secretary. I have   attached two documents -the first is where I was up to with organisers etc and the other is the updated results spreadsheet (NB ladies results not linked to the VTTA standards, but men have the new standards in place). For the Novice event Maurice agreed to time keep for both events and John L agreed to help at one of these.

John

From: John Bosley **Subject:** Re: TT documents
To: "richard n" **Date:** Wednesday, 6 March, 2013, 10:41

Thanks Dick.

Kate is now out of intensive care and her life-threatening situation is now stable. I guess it's just a day at a time now to see what she can re-learn. She has significant brain damage and they are struggling to know exactly what the long term effects of this will be, mobility, cognitive, senses?

Thanks, John

From: richard n **Sent:** 06 March 2013 16:45
To: John Bosley **Subject:** Re: TT documents

Let's hope for more good news John, our thoughts are with Kate, willing for a full recovery.

Take care Dick

From: John Bosley **Sent:** Wednesday, March 06, 2013 6:38 PM
To: Bernard Wilson **Subject:** Repatriation?

Hi,

I spoke with the insurers and repatriation may be sooner than expected ... They even suggested that one of you may be able to escort her back! They have to finalise a bed, which hasn't been done yet. They will need Kate's passport info from you as well. You may want to look at www.airmed.co.uk though I don't promise that's them!

One insurer has asked for a document from the hospital. Something that proves where she was and for what period of time. Such as a discharge letter. Not sure how easy that will be but good if they offer it!

I've had some unpleasant communications with the firm that manage the house in Southwold! They have refused any refund for the weekend which I felt was poor in the circumstances.

Looking forward to hearing about Kate today!
John

From: Bernard   **Sent:** 06 March 2013 21:11
To: John Bosley   **Subject:** Re: Repatriation?
Hi John,

Yes, I had this info from the insurers too about them flying out here tomorrow and returning with Kate and possibly Janet on Friday. It would have to be Janet, I couldn't leave her here alone! That will mess up the Annie meeting arrangements, but I'll sort that out. One snag as you will have read in my text, the hospital are not aware of these plans! They will have to get together with the insurers asap if they are to fly the air ambulance out tomorrow. I can't do anything, although I am waiting for a call from the insurers now, they want passport details and they were locked in the safe when they rang me on the way to the hospital.

How is Kathy? Brighter every day, more movement, more energy, but there still is the communication problem. She moves her lips but we can't read what she is saying or asking. I tried my new communication board which Janet had made, but she wouldn't even point to the yes and no "buttons". The nurse had brought her a white board and a marker and asked her to write. She didn't want to, but when the nurse insisted she produced a scribble. Of course, her right hand is affected, though she can now do a light squeeze. I didn't pursue the experiment, it seemed unkind. She was happy holding my hand and listening to Miss Saigon. Once she pulled my hand to her face and kissed it! We don't know what damage there is in the cognitive area, she may be temporarily unable to discriminate shapes and letters, and doesn't want us to know that she doesn't recognise alphabetic characters. She knows where she is, she knows she has had an accident, but she is puzzled about it. I thought it best to leave the full details for you to impart in due course.

Just spoken to the insurers. The arrangements are to fly from Tenerife North at 8.00am arriving Biggin Hill at 3.30pm and then ambulance to Maidstone hospital!

What do you think of that!

I look forward to your comments,

So happy for you, Kathy and the kids,

Love from B&J

From: John Bosley   **Sent:** Wednesday, March 06, 2013 10:23 PM

To: Bernard **Subject:** Re: Repatriation?

All a bit of a rush! What does Janet think about travelling in the air ambulance? I think I may stay at home in the morning (at least!) and make some calls to chase things!

It's good news about Kate. It can be a little worrying to think too much about what she can't do. I'm trying my best to think about what she can do and believe that she will continue to progress and if necessary re-learn things and allow her brain to make new connections.

I hope she isn't so different when she comes out at the other end.

It looks like your trip to Tenerife has a clearer finish?!

Love John   Sent from my iPad

On 7 Mar 2013, at 19:50, "Bernard" wrote:

Dear John,

This will be brief because we have to be up early and we haven't eaten all day! We have spent 4 hours with Kathy and have left her with Nikky and Phil. They arrived just as we were thinking of leaving. As I told you, Kathy is now breathing normally. It takes a bit of getting used to, and speech came slowly, but it was good to hear her talking at last even if it was difficult to follow sometimes. She is worrying about her work, and about the American holiday. We tried to put her mind at rest, but were pleased that she came up with these problems on her own, she clearly has no memory problems about future plans. Of course, she remembers nothing about being in IC, the family's visits, or the incident which caused all this. I don't think she remembers why she is in Tenerife either. I told her that so many people were asking after her, and she wanted to know who! So I mentioned names including Annie, Roger, Marianna, and all these names were significant to her.

Everything should be OK for a 7:00am ambulance trip to the airport, plane leaving at 8:00 and due at Biggin Hill at 3:30pm. I suppose she will be at Maidstone by 4:30ish. Will there be someone to let Jan in? Alan will be picking her up between 7:00 and 8:00 on his way down from Derbyshire. She will spend the night with them and he will take her home on Saturday. That's all worked out very well!

I am going to try to get her flight changed to my name and then brought forward a day or two.

Must go now, so glad to be bringing this news, which seemed an impossible dream a week ago!

Love from B&J

From: John Bosley   **Sent:** Thursday, March 07, 2013 8:22 PM

To: Bernard   **Subject:** Re: Repatriation?

Blimey, that sounds amazing! I have been on the phone to Maidstone Assessment unit to see if I can be there when Kate arrives. Will Janet be with her at that point? If not Josh is at Uni until about 5.30pm on a Friday but Sarah usually gets home by 4pm.

(By the way, that's a long flight time ... Do they carry enough fuel?).

Changing the name? Moving the flight? That will probably cost more than booking a new flight (to the moon), Good luck!

I've doubted all week coming home. It's been good to get Sarah and Josh back to 'school', to sort out some business etc but it's been uncomfortable. Kate coming back this quick is fantastic.

Love John

From: Bernard   **Sent:** 07 March 2013 21:16
To: John Bosley   **Subject:** Re: Repatriation?

We assume that Janet will travel with Kathy to Maidstone since she will have been with her all day but who knows?

Must start booking...............................

Love Bernard

From: alisonm   **Sent:** 07 March 2013 21:10 **To:** jbosley **Subject:** Kate

Hi John

Just to let you know how pleased we are that Kathy is on the way home - that sounds really lame - actually we are much more than pleased!!!. It is great news. Do let us know if there is anything at all that we can do. Are her mum and dad coming back with her?

I will try to come and see her one weekend soon when she is settled in the hospital. Is she likely to stay in Maidstone Hospital?

Saw that Sarah did really well today too so congrats to her!

You must have been brilliant to keep everyone going too!

Take Care Ali

PS Jo and Yam send their love - Sarah has been keeping Beth up to date

From: Dave S **Sent:** 07 March 2013 20:21 **To:** J Bosley **Subject:** Kate
Hi John

I'm really glad to hear Kate is making progress and will back here tomorrow. I can't begin to imagine all you are going through but I'd like to send Kate all my best wishes for her full recovery - there's not been a day gone by since I heard of her accident that I haven't thought of you all and what you are going through.

PS No need for you to reply you have more important things to deal with.
Dave
(David is a friend)

From: David B **Sent:** 07 March 2013 21:00 **To:** J Bosley **Subject:** Kate
Hi John

I'm shocked and really sorry to hear about Kate. (You're right I am not a Facebook user so this is the first news!) Please send my best wishes to Kate and wish her a speedy recovery. Let me know if I can help in anyway. I am feeling for you mate, not easy at the best of times, let alone in a different country. Thanks for the update.
Take care   David

From: Nicola and Philip K **Sent:** 07 March 2013 23:13
To: john bosley **Subject:** RE: Kate
Hi John

Just back from our visit to Kate. Thanks for the helpful info about finding the hospital and parking, it was indeed a nightmare and so badly sign posted! Bernard met us and filled us in a bit then he and Janet headed home. We were around when the doctor and nurse from the air ambulance came to assess Kate so hopefully that was helpful. They both seemed lovely and will ensure Kate has as good a trip home as possible. I warned them of her fear of flying and if necessary they will provide some sedation. She was so much better than we expected and seems to be coming on in leaps and bounds. She was talking well and getting clearer as we spent more time listening and as she practised. The trachy had been capped in the afternoon so she hadn't been speaking for long.

Typically she was worrying about everyone else but was aware she needed to be a good patient and be thinking about her needs. I managed to help her with some yoghurt.

We will be in touch when we get home
love Nicky and Phil

From: "Bernard" **Date:** 7 March 2013 22:11:41 **To:** Roger M **Subject:** Kate

Dear Roger,

I'm assuming that you have been kept up to date with the news, so I'll get straight to the latest. Kate is coming home tomorrow by air ambulance. She will be brought by ambulance from Biggin Hill to Maidstone Hospital, arriving late afternoon (Friday 8th). Janet is travelling with her, so I have cancelled her flight. I will be arriving Heathrow 18:50 on Saturday (Iberia from Madrid). So please tell Annie she will not be needed after all! But many thanks.

I will take the train from Heathrow via London, so no problem!

Kate had her tracheostomy tube capped today and was breathing normally and at   last able to talk. She has a clear memory of the past and of future plans (her trip to America) but does not know where she is or how she got there. I have told her enough to satisfy her I think. She understands that you have all been thinking of her and sending good wishes, I mentioned you, Annie and Marianna and she smiled in recognition and thanks.

It's been tough for us all, but it's reached this stage so much sooner than we could have dared to hope. Thank you so much for your support!

I hope that we will meet sometime soon,

Best wishes, Bernard and Janet

From: Bernard **Sent:** 08 March 2013 08:26
To: J Bosley **Subject:** At last!

Dear John,

By now they should be on their way! I tried to get a photo of Kathy being loaded into the ambulance but was sternly rebuked by the driver! Kathy is so much better this-morning, even from last night. She is talking, and showing concern for the "trouble" she has caused! We talked about the family and I asked her what she thought Sarah would do when she finished her education. Kathy said "She'll be brilliant at anything!" That shows how far she has come in a week!

Janet was asking anxiously about the flight. She was told that the aircraft is very small, there is not even a toilet on board! They will land in Portugal to refuel and for toilet needs. Poor Janet paled at this news, but I said "You must be strong for Katy!" Easy for me to say that! The nurse assured me that both would be sedated if necessary. There is a nurse and doctor travelling in the plane, they both saw Kate yesterday just after we had left, and they said that there was a marked improvement today. I think 4 hours with us and probably 2 with the Kings had worn her out!

The ambulance left with all lights flashing and horns sounding! That was the last I saw of them. Now for breakfast! Hope you get to see Kathy tonight OK. What a change you will see!

Bye,

Love Bernard

On 8 Mar 2013, at 08:21, Roger M wrote:
Dear John,
This is indeed great news! Wishing you all well with the move today and I look forward to catching up with you over the weekend. When you see Kate send her the love and best wishes of all her friends and colleagues at the Hospice. We very much look forward to seeing her ourselves!
Best wishes, Roger

On 8 Mar 2013, at 08:25, John Bosley wrote:
Thanks Roger, sounds like amazing and exciting progress.
John

On 8 Mar 2013, at 21:21, Roger M wrote:
Hi John,
Well, how did things go? Have been thinking about you both all day. Fingers crossed.
Best wishes, Roger

On 8 Mar 2013, at 23:01, John Bosley wrote:
Just got back! She has arrived safely and is in the assessment unit for now. Tomorrow I'll sneak in late morning and see if I can be with her as she gets moved to a ward. Her progress is amazing Roger but there are significant problems for her to overcome ... Hopefully given time. We had a lovely 4 or 5 hours together though.
John

From: Roger M **Sent:** 08 March 2013 23:09
To: John Bosley **Subject:** Re: Kate

Wonderful news!

I will catch up with you over the weekend. Kate must be exhausted after her long journey today. But I'm sure she is pleased to be home.

Best wishes Roger

On 9 Mar 2013, at 13:52, John Bosley wrote:

Kate is on Whatman Ward temporarily. They want her on another rehab.ward where she can get daily physio etc but because she has a trachy she is on Whatman to begin with. The Drs will review her trachy on Monday and expect to remove it. They will also remove her cannula now.

Visiting is between 3 and 5 pm and 6.30 - 7.30. Apart from us I will encourage people in a few days to contact me if they wish to visit. I've already had about 10 requests and it'll waste people's time if they arrive and someone is already there, more importantly will be no good for Kate.

Kate has come on amazingly but there are some key difficulties for her that I have witnessed:

1. She is now able to squeeze her right hand but not lift her right arm. If holding hands etc concentrate on her right hand/arm!

2. She uses the wrong words regularly which mean some things don't make sense ... If you have no idea what she is saying please do not be condescending and pretend you understand. Just make a good guess and then check with her if you got it right. Apologise if you can't work it out!

3. She has a tendency to give the wrong answer, either to please people or because she doesn't know. eg. Asked if she wants tea or coffee, she asked for coffee possibly because it was the last thing said. Then, with milk "yes" with sugar "yes". Kate doesn't take it with sugar. (Let's not argue for the minute over whether her tastes have changed!)

4. She is inconsistent with her memory. At the moment she does not know that she is the CEO of a hospice ... unless prompted.

5. She is far too nice. Worrying about others around her, telling the nurses what a good job they are doing (they are) etc. but I don't think she fully comprehends her situation. I had explained a couple of times that we were going to a ward. When I asked her where are we going now, she answered 'Home?' I'd love to think that was a joke ...

There's lots more, but her progress is stunning so let's help her to improve with these things over the coming weeks!

John

PS I'm pleased to say she knows who I am! She said, "Will you come back soon, John?" and leant over to give me a good-bye kiss (coughing and depositing some phlegm on my upper lip!). You can't help but love her!

On 9 Mar 2013, at 14:18, Cheryl W wrote:

Hi John

Thanks so much for the update. Please can Alan and I visit next Saturday (Alan will be back down next weekend from Derbyshire) ....3pm would be good if that fits in with the rest of the family. Take care and send our love to Kathryn in the meantime.

Lots of love Cheryl and Alan Xx

From: JohnB **To:** cheryl
Sent: 9 Mar 2013 14:22 **Subject:** Whatman Ward

Yes that'd be fine. We'll need to keep in contact about which ward she is on.   PS. You're not on Facebook are you?

From: cheryl   **Sent:** 9 March 2013 14:27
To: JohnB **Subject:** Whatman Ward

Hi John

Thanks that's great. If you could let us know the ward nearer the time that'd be great. Sorry not on Facebook!

You take care xx

From: Bernard   **Sent:** 09 March 2013 19:53
To: John Bosley **Subject:** Re: Whatman Ward

Thanks for those helpful observations. I want to see her ASAP but won't be home till late tonight. I'll contact you tomorrow about visiting.

Bernard

All this over less than 3 weeks and it's only a selection! It was so lovely to know people cared but it ended up a full time job making sure I responded.

THE CHILDREN'S BOOK PART 1

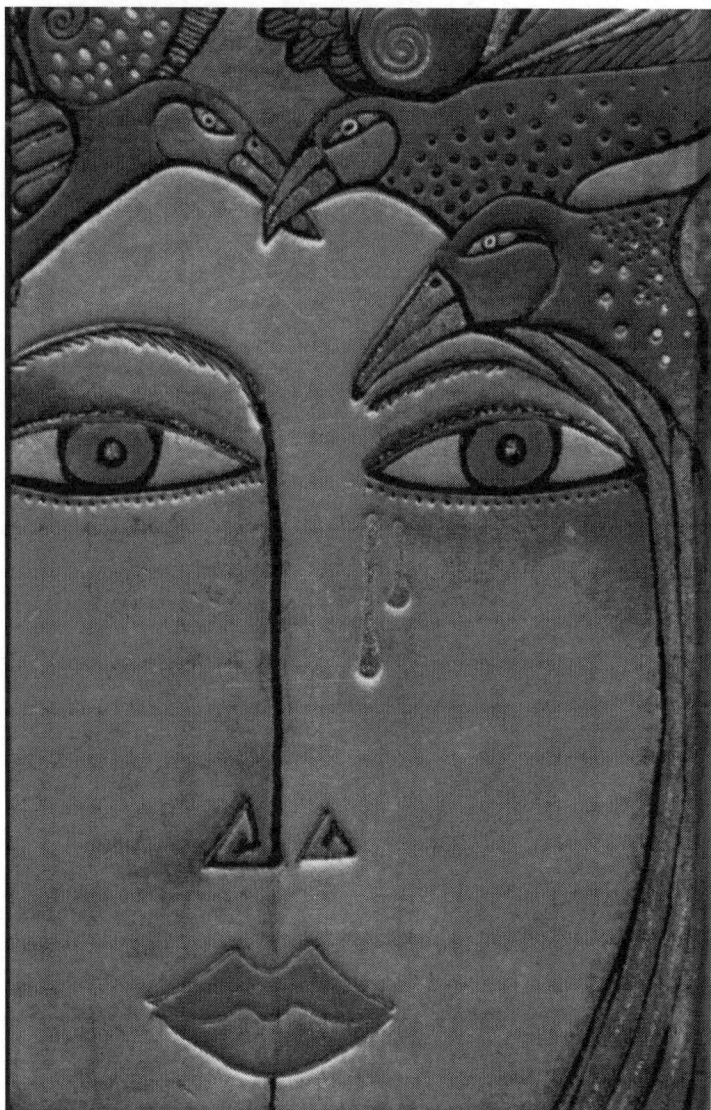

Hannah   24/2/13
_____

Hi, Mum,   Josh and I have
been here since Friday now
we came to visit on ~~Satud~~
Friday at 6pm. luckily we were
very early as we thought it was 7pm.
Dad had explained that you were
completly still since monday
but whilst we visited we saw
you open your eyes, stretch your
legs and Josh saw you yawn!.
The longuoge barrier is a
bit of a problem so we are
Just guessing what all this
means.
The insurance doctor will ring
today so hopefully we will
have a better understanding.
I have written a poem for
you.

.

26/02/13

It's me again!
I came to visit you at 1:00 today and you seemed to move quite a bit. Obviously my presence is over powering! Haha. As Hannah said before, your swelling has gone so we're all very happy about that! Now we just need you to wake up.. C'mon Mum!

The doctors say you're not responding to their orders e.g "squeeze my hand" however you never did enjoy being bossed around.

All my friends are going crazy at school apparantly. hopfully now Miss. Sosimi will go easy on me. ☺

I love you Mum

Sarah xxxxxx

27/4/13

went to see you again today
I asked you to do a Back flip
but you didn't! however you were
unable before the accident so it
was a bit of a long shot!!
found a shopping centre and
had a lovely meal, Josh
XXXXX

Sarah,

Last night me and Charlotte arrived in Tenerife (24/02/18) The flight was good however we had to fly from Heathrow to Madrid (2½ hours) and then from Madrid to Tenerife (2½ hours.) It was OK though. We had a great McDonalds at the airport! We were greeted by Hannah, Josh and Dad but then discovered Iberia had lost our luggage. Not good.

Later on today I will visit you for the first time, I'm a little bit apprehensive but very excited.

P.S. Skiing was amazing!

Hannah   24/2/13
_____

Hi mum,   Josh and I have
been here since Friday now
we came to visit on ~~Satur~~
Friday at 6pm. luckily we were
very early as we thought it was 7pm.
Dad had explained that you were
completly still since monday
but whilst we visited we saw
you open your eyes, stretch your
legs and Josh saw you yawn!.
The language barrier is a
bit of a problem so we are
just guessing what all this
means.
The insurance doctor will ring
today so hopefully we will
have a better understanding.
I have written a poem for
you.

My mum

I got the call on the 20th Feb
The day my life turned on its head
"Mum's been in a coma for 3 days"
So now we're all in a bit of a daze

By friday we were on our flight
and im trying to stay strong
with all my might.
In Tenerife we found somewhere to stay
Just 20 mins from from where mum lay.

Visiting times for just 1 hour
you want to do more but have no power
She's as beautiful as ever but its a
scary sight
Though we can see already mums
putting up a fight

A bit of a back story
for you all to see
my mum is simply
the best there can be!
Its as simple as that,
there is no other
we are so lucky to have our mother.

Though the hospital is a bit of a
botch
The room and equipment looks top
notch. .
The language barrier is not ideal
and with no information it
doesn't seem real!

a blink and a kick is
enough to excite
wee thinking movement is good,
right?
My sisters will join us today (day 3)
and hopefully there will be more to see!
Mum is strong and so are we!
Soon, um sure she'll be home for
tea!

Love you mum! xxxxxxxx
               xxxxxxxx
                x infinity...

                  25/2/13
  you look good today! (everyone says
  you look more like me!) Was very hot and
  we had a Subway so good day! :)
  xxxxxxx

179

Mummy!!

I wish I yes knew more about intensive care so I could tell everyone exactly what was happening but Hannah had figured out all the bits I knew anyway before me and Sarah arrived e.g you are being NG fed. (Sean is now moaning cause he says he worked it out as well)

I'm surprised how good you look with a shaved head although they missed a few annoying strands that make you look Jewish.

We hope we have more of an update about whats

happening tommorrow. And
some more movement from
you would be lovely
bubbly.
    Love you massively
                Charlotte
                    xxxx

Saw you for the first time
today. You still look beautiful
bald somehow? You looked
very peaceful which made
me feel better. Your food
looked like Chocolate milk
which I know you wouldn't
be to impressed about. I half
expected there to be tomatoes
floating around just for you.
Your bed looks top knotch

by the way, a lot comfier than mine and Charlottes large plank of wood.
I love you to infinity and beyond, xxxxxxx
x x x x x x x

Sarah :)

Hannah   26/2/13

Hi mum,
We came to see you at lunch
time today in the hope that we
would be able to speak to
a Doctor.
Charlotte, Sarah and dad were there
when the Doctor came into the
room.
Apparently the doctor had
said the swelling has gone
down which is good!
However we were told that
you were not sedated and
as we saw little movement
that was pretty scary!
We had already expected this
would be a long process so
I have planned to come
back out here with Sarah

During the easter holiday. Hopefully we will have a little longer to plan it this time. The doctor also asked dad to sign something to give the permission to give you a Tracheostomy.

I have googled it all but the answer/outcome is completely individual so I guess we just have to wait and see.

We all love you lots! xxxxx
P.S I got an email from the human resources dept at Cancer research.
They said they think my skill sets would suit a community fundraising role in Essex.

I know you would advise
me to stay at Richard House
and I dont fancy moving
just yet anyway.
Still, its nice to know
youre wanted isnt it.
lots of love!
xxxxxx
Hannah
xxxxx

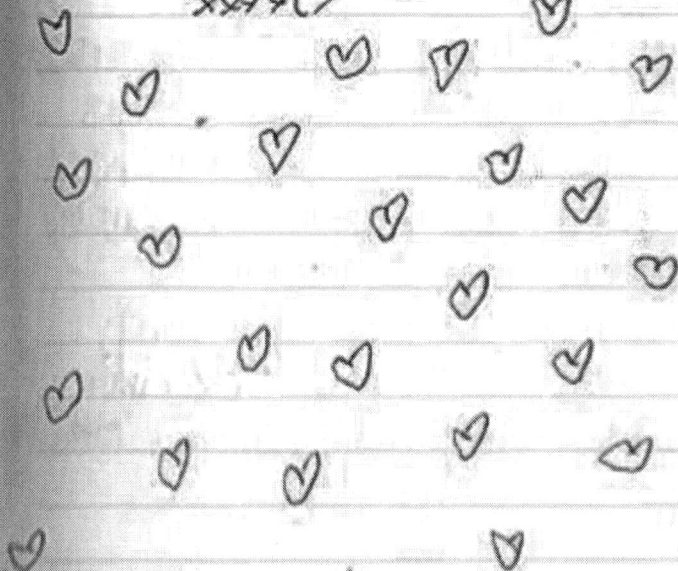

26/02/13

It's me again!
I came to visit you at 1:00 today and you seemed to move quite a bit. Obviously my presence is over powering! Haha. As Hannah said before, your swelling has gone so we're all very happy about that! Now we just need you to wake up... C'mon Mum!

The doctors say you're not responding to their orders e.g "squeeze my hand" how-ever you never did enjoy being bossed around.

All my friends are going crazy at school apparantly. hopefully now Miss. Sosimi will go easy on me. :)

I love you Mum

Sarah xxxxx

27/2/13

Hannah here,

Today was a good day Considering
the situation.
We went to a Museum which
was really impressive! we also
went to the "Sydney" oprah house
well at least it looked like it.
there were lots of rocks going
out to sea with graffiti on them.
I will show you a picture.
We also ate at a really nice/
cheap resturante then we
came to see you again.
We played you music and
when i was in the room
me and Charlie played and
sang james blunt and you
seemed to respond to this.

you moved your arm a
few times and moved your
lips too! ♡
The insurange company said ♡
they are thinking about
trying to get you back home
which means you will have
to take an air Ambulanse.
Hopefully this will be ♡
less scary for you.
If they are sensible they won't
tell you you are about to fly.
Josh and I have to go
home soon, which is sad!
I cant wait for you to
come home so I can visit
if not, i will come back
here soon!
lots of love
♡   Hannah xy

27/02/13

Today we did something with our day and visited a museum. It was nicer than moping around! After that and grabbing a bite to eat we came to see you again. I feel quite proud of myself as I seem to be dealing with this a lot better than the other wimps at the hospital. One man went in to his relatives room and came straight back out crying. You've obviously brought us up right! Not going to lie... I have cried alot but I try not to cry in front of you as I don't want to scare you, however Charlie did set me off today whilst we played you a bit of Les Mis. You didn't seem to like that much but you had a bit of a jig to James Blunt!

We got a call from the Insurers today and they mensioned flying you home which would be amazing as we might actually be able to understand what's going on!

Please wake up soon because people are starting to worry... hahaha. Love you so much.
Sazbomb
xxxxxxx

28th February 2013

Hiya mum
        Today when we visited
you had already had your
tracheostomy inserted
which we all liked because
it means we could see
your face a lot better
as you now only have
a nasogastric tube in
and there was another tube
going through the same
nostril but I couldn't work
out what it was for. was it
Seems to be attached to
a monitor so I was unsure
if it was monitoring
CO_2 or something.

I gave the nurses chocolate
and a post card which
said "Gracias por cuidas
de mi mama" which hopefully
means "thank you for looking
after my mum" but god
only knows what it says
as I had googled it but
the nursing staff seemed
quite happy and thankful.
      Granny + Grandad
are coming tomorrow and
Nikki King is visiting
soon which I think you
will love.
      Josh + Hannah have
to go back to UK
tommorow. so hopefully
you will give us some more
more ment tomoz
      I love you so so much
                        Charliebean

"You've been the greatest
mother to me,
Teaching me many things
that others never see,
And so I write to you
this very day
And hope my love will
bless you in every way."

Today you didn't do much
... BORING! You were on
Morphine so probably pretty
sleepy. Charlotte told you
she loved you and you
moved alot and then went
still again, that was nice.
I really miss you mum.
I love you like crazy.

Love Sarah xxxxx

28th ~ Hannah

Tomorrow Josh and I
have to leave. We are
not sure what will happen
in the near future but
I will take two weeks off
at easter and spend it
with you whereever you are.
Today you didnt move much
Charlie wonderd if that
was because you were on
morphine.
hopefully we will have
more luck tomorrow (our
last day).
Everyone is asking about
you. Even some of the
newspapers. We are all
constantly answering emails/
texts etc constantly!!!

Dad spoke to J9
today, he seemed to
completly understand
what was going on and
he showed a lot of
concern.
Grandma Grumps and
Grandad will come
tomorrow so you will
have someone with you
as much as the hospital
will allow,
Nicki king is also going
to visit you soon so
thats something to look
forward to.
It seems strange that i
cant just ring you for
a chat,
your a strong woman mum!
We love you lots! xx

I have got to remember to
stop feeling sorry for myself.
Your the one fighting for
your life!
Plus some people dont have
any hope if thier loved ones
pass away straight away following
an accident.
We have lots of hope.
Your the most amazing
woman in the world if
anyone can do it, you can!
xxx
love you so much! xxx

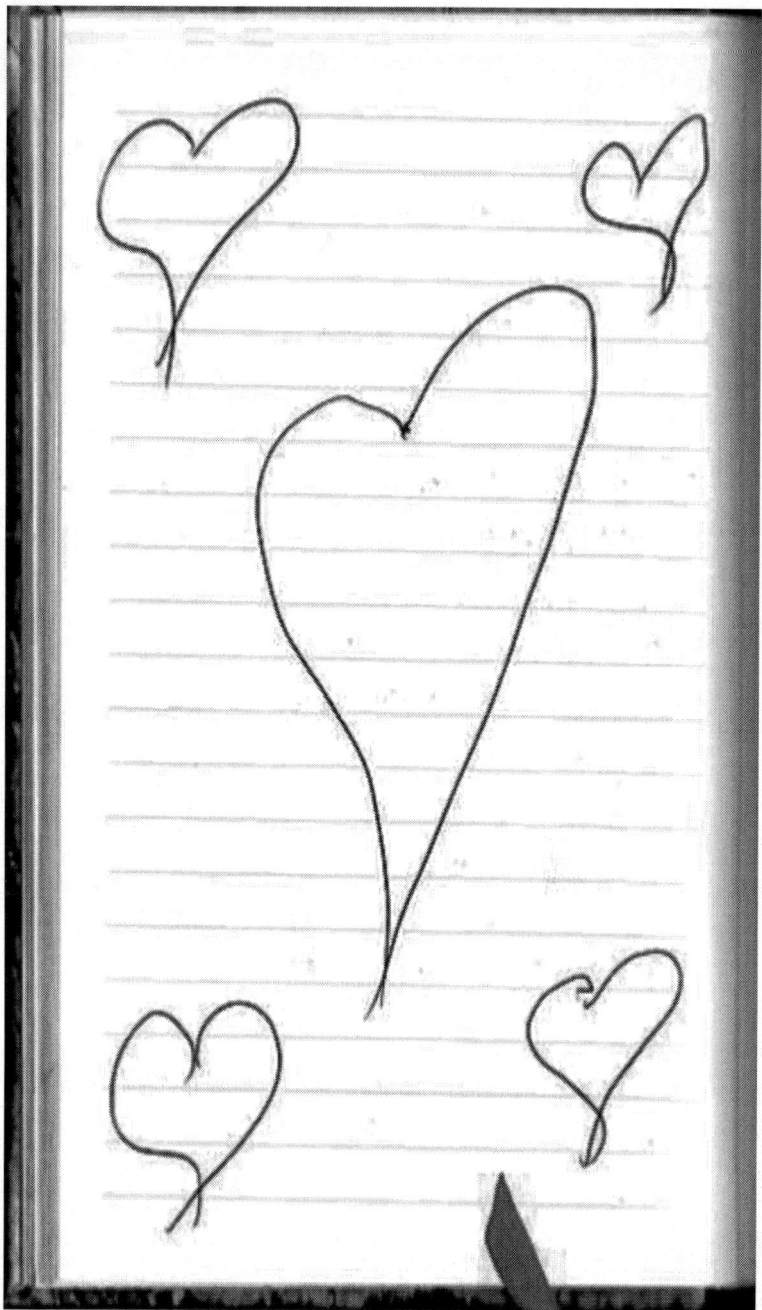

1/3/13

New Month, New hope!!

We were so happy that when we saw you today you were conscious!! I grabbed your hand and asked you to squeeze my hand and you squeezed and squeezed and squeezed I have never been sooo happy.

I know you know we are all there and even smiled at some saves and remarks but you also looked scared I think I tried to reassure you that you were sore and that

everything was going to
be OK!! You must be
so scared!!!

I wish we could
sit with you all day
but the visiting times
are very strict.

Grandma + grandad arrived
this evening and we took
them straight to the
hospital after telling them
of your improvement.

You were still conscious
and doing the same sort
of things although you
looked exhausted!! I think
you had had a tough
day!!!

Cant wait to see

you tomorrow we will visit twice however I will be very sad as it will be our last visit as my flight home is Sunday!!

I'm hoping sooo much that we will be able to fly you home ASAP so I can visit as often as is possible.

I love you so much and told you that many times over the last few days.

I hope you heard me and understood me todays and remember it when I have to leave.

Keep Fighting love Charlotte xx

1st March 2013

Today I walked into your room and expected you to be lying in your bed unconscious like you have been for almost 2 weeks but today was different. I walked in to see you looking at me and not only were you conscious you were breathing by yourself!

You're on the road to recovery and I am so proud of you. There's a long way to go but we all believe in you.

Tomorrow will be my last day which is sad but I am so glad I got to

see your improvements!
I love you like crazy
Mum,
Sarah xxxxx

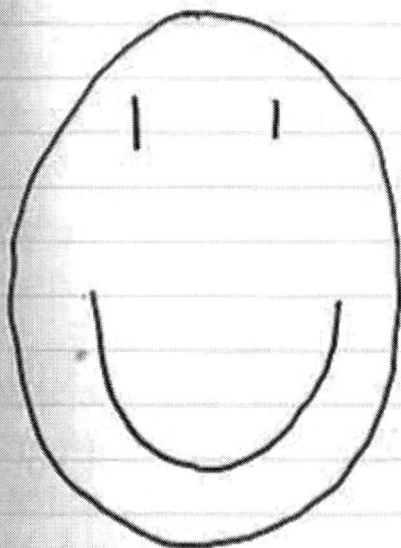

HANNAH

Hi mum, I haven't had
the book so I haven't been
able to write in it for a
few days.

The last time I wrote to you
you were still in a coma and
you had just had your tracheostomy
operation.

Friday was our last day (me and
Sash) so we were really anxious
to see some improvement before
we left you.

Sarah went in to intensive care
first and came out straight
away waving for someone to take
her place. I swopped with her
wondering what all the fuss
was about. When I walked
in you looked straight at me
and smiled!

I got very excited and congratulated you and you smiled again.
Dad said kathy you have had any crash and you raised your eyebrows as if to say "well obviously" you were also squeezing our hands when we asked you to and I told you Josh wasn't impressed, he was hoping for a backflip. Josh said, you don't have to do it now, maybe tomorrow and you laughed at this

I stupidly asked you what your fav food was as we couldn't get into your bank and you looked as if you were really trying to tell us. It looked hard work so we told you not to worry.

I have never been so happy in all my life!

You were in a coma for 12 days and now your awake.

Charlotte had brought some chocolates and a card for the Neuro staff the day before. He card said 'thank you for looking after my mummy. (we think).

We joke that the bribe had worked and now the nurses are working even harder on you.

Hi mum!!

We visited you this morning and saw your Dr he is very nice and speaks good english. He basically said you had weakness on your ℗ side that would need physio but they expect it to get better in the future with lots of effort.

You were asleep when we visited today I think you were exhausted after your first day conscious and self ventilating yesterday!

Although you were asleep you gave some amazing hand squeezing and some wild leg movements!!

At one point I had to save your urinary catheter as you were really pulling on it. I think its really irritating you.

The doctor also said you were ready to be moved onto a ward there you could have more input in terms of physio and nursing input which would be really good although we think you won't be in Tenerife for too long.

The doctors say they are updating the insurers and letting them no what equipment is needed to safely transfer you home.

Today was my last visit until I had to go home. At lunch time you were asleep but you grabbed my hand and wouldn't let go which is comforting. This evening you were asleep again (I don't blame you) but your arm and leg was strapped to the bed, I guess you were being stubborn and trying to pull your catheter out. Hopefully you won't need it for much longer. It was tough leaving you today but I know you're in safe hands and we're hoping you will be air ambulanced home soon, if not I will definitely

See you at Easter.
I go back to school on
Monday (all my mocks)
great! But I'm looking
forward to it.

I Love You sooo much.
Seriously.
Get well soon!
Sarah
x x x x x
x x x x x
x x x x x

♡

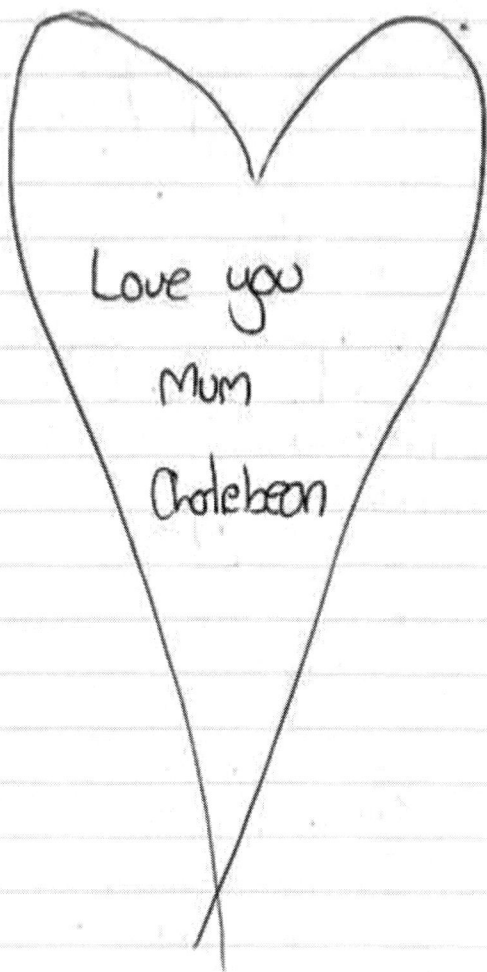

Love you

Mum

Chotebean

4/3/13

Ok!! So I've been
thinking this is all
very confusing so
conted to do myself
a quick timeline!

Monday 18th February 2013
= You have a bike
accident. We don't know
what happened!!!

= You are now in a coma
and intubated.

Wednesday 20th February 2013
= Still intubated Dad
phones us and tells us
you are in intensive care
in tenerife intubated
Sarah is saying and doesn't
know

Friday 22nd February 2013
= Hannah + Josh fly
out to Tenerife. They
get to visit you
you are still unconscious
and intubated.

Saturday 23rd February 2013
= Sarah returns from
Skiing I have to
tell her the bad news

Sunday 24th February 2013
= Me + Sarah fly out
to Tenerife we arrive
to late to see you
but you are still
unconscious + intubated

Wednesday 27th February 2013
= Still unconscious +
Intubated Doctors
say it will be better
for you to have a
tracheostomy. Dad
gave them signed consent
today.

Thursday 28th February 2013
= Tracheostomy inserted
Still unconscious +
intubated -

Friday 1st March 2013
= Suddenly you are
conscious and self
ventilating via tracheostomy
obeying commands making
eye contact!.. xx

Cant believe it?!! Soah
+ honah have to leave
grodma + grondad arived

Saturday 2nd Morch 2013
⇒ You slept both
visits But Doctor
Said you were still
progressing Just tired.

Sunday 3rd Morch 2013
⇒ Me, Soah + Dad had
to leave but grondad
Says you were being
spoon Fed AMAZING!!

Monday 4th Morch 2013
Grondad hasn't Given
any update yet but I
miss you and hope

214

insurers will fly
us you back ASAP!!

P.S. Our Goal is for you
to make it to USA
with us so get
re-learning.

love Charliebean.

update

Monday 4th March 2013
- You have been moved
to a rehab ward
your taking small amounts
off of a spoon
Amaze walls!!!

215

Thursday 7th March 2013
= Been hard keeping
up to date with your
progress not being in
theatre. But the aim
is to fly you home
tomorrow.
Can't wait to see you
Grandad seems to
say they have blocked/
removed your trache
ad your starting to
talk.
Grandad says your
worried about Florida
don't worry

WE WILL GO TO
FLORIDA
I promise.

Hannah

over the past (week
I flew back from tenerife
stayed with Auntie sarah
and met up with G-dad Boz
and sue. ~~crutton~~ Everyone
was very sopportive!
I went to work and it
was quite difficult because
really um thinking about
you the whole time.
Everyone is asking how you
are and its really hard
because i don't know
what the answer is.
we have had daily updates
from grandad and we hear
that you can talk now
he says that you mentioned
florida but its hard to
imagine as we havent seen

it for ourselves.
I found out that you will be flown home on Friday (8th) which is just in time for mothers day and your birthdays!
I am a bit nurvous about coming to visit because I am afraid you would not lonow who we are. but at the same time I can't wait to see you again.
We love you so so much and whilst it seems a coincidence that I would end up having the best mum in the world.
Coincidences Happen! and we are so so luckly. xxx
lots of love Hannah xx

Sat 9th March - Hannah

We came to visit you at maidstone today. you were sitting with old people and charlotte pointed out that you were in the wrong ward.

but hopefully you will be moved somewhere nicer and safer.

We came to visit you at about 3 today. You were wide eyed and spoke quite clearly. Most of what you told us made some sense as Charlotte said.

you said started to name us all "Charlotte, Hannah, Joshua ..... and after a breath you said Sarah" that was quite tense because for a split second we thought you had forgotton Sarah's name. you said that you had been fine but today you thought you had been naughty. Before you thought you had been told off. the nurse looked a bit worried and reassured you that you were not in trouble. she then went on to tell us that one of the nurses came across quite abrupt because she was from portuagal. Mainly you seemed to worry about work you wanted us to bring your timetable in you also worried about your weight which is typical you!, and you were worried about other ~~patients~~ patients in the ward. Again, typical you! when me and charlie came to say goodbye we asked you if you wanted us to bring something, we offered to bring in some food or a film and you said a film because then we wouldent be bored watching you.

Its mothers day tomorrow and we are looking forward to coming to visit!

lots of love xy

Hannah xx

10th March 2013

I can't believe the extent of your progress. Last time I saw you you were not very aware of your surroundings and couldn't talk. Today I walked in and you said hello and smiled. We had a lovely chat but you were exhausted. It was nice to just sit and talk, you don't make perfect sense sometimes but when I think about it I understand what you're trying to say.

It was lovely to see you and I will be coming every day after school.

Love you millions
Sarah xxxxxxx

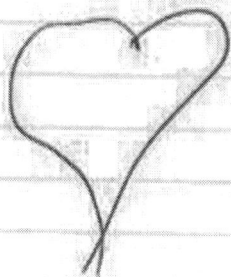

Monday 11th March 2013

Mummy today was your birthday you are 100% convinced your 21 I have to keep telling you your 51 and you pull the funniest face when I tell you that says "oh dear, thats not good".

Shoila made you cupcakes and your reaction was amazing you ate an entire cupcake (you haven't been eating much).

I made you get out of bed and sit in a chair today which was good progress. Walking tomorow!!!

love charliebean

Hannah - 11th March

We came to visit again yesterday
and it was mothers day.
You seemed happy to see us.
I showed you some photographs
and you managed to point out
our immediate family but
you struggled to remember
new people like Simon.
thought i can see recognition
on your face, think your just
getting confused with names.
Though you can answer questions
like "what do you want to eat"
most of the time it makes
sense its just not what we would
expect for example you ask for
sugar in your tea and we
know that you would not
normally have sugar.

However occasionally you will
say something completely
irrelevant like
"what do you want to drink"
and you would answer
"January"..
today is your Birthday and
i can't wait for Charlotte to
collect me and take me
to visit you!
oh she is here now!
see you soon

Hannah x

12th March 2013

So today I arrived
with bash to find
you clombering out of
the end of the bed inbetween
the bars and the foot
end. The nuse said the
occupational therapist
took you for a walk
earlier on in the morning
and now you think you
can just get up and
walk anymore even
though your very coddely
(you did have a little
well when we got there)
    Anyway the occupational
therapist Serah has
refered you to a
neuro rehab unit in

227

Sevenoaks which sounds really good and much better for you.

I hope you don't try and do any walking without help overnight because you will fall and its really worrying one.

Tommorow is my last day in maidstone so i'll come and visit before netball. Then I won't see you for a little while until I come back.

But I think that you will be busy loads of people wanna visit.

love Charlie Bson

Wednesday 13th March 203

Hi Mum.

Came to visit today. Sally Furlong came to visit and gave you a slice of cake which you ate all of (the lady said you hadn't eaten your lunch so you must of been hungry)

The lovely healthcare assistant and Occupational therapist said you had been for a really long walk and had gone on on exercise bike!) amazing!) You only got out of bed for a little while for the first time on Monday!

The health care assistant said you had told her you had 3 daughters and 1 Son and one of your daughters went to valley forge!

Thats amazing memory. I'm so impressed.

I'm going back to Lochloiheoad tonight so won't see you for a little while.

I know you will have 100° of visitors though!

They are. Still hoping to have you referred to a neuro rehab centre in Sevenoaks.

Dad told you Roger is visiting tomorrow and he

asked you if you knew who Roger was and you said "My boss" so we really are getting better.

Also I asked you how old you were and instead of your usual '21' response you said '45' so we are getting there.

Love you very much

Charlie bean

X X X x X

Hannah   13th March

Hi Mum,
me and charlotte came to visit
on monday (your 51st Birthday)
we saw lots of improvements
and we even got you out
of your bed and into the chair.
You were convinced you were
21 though and you forgot
my name a few times.
We Brought you your Lucky
charm thomas Jatso Birthday
Present and you liked it but
you were even more impressed
with Sheila's cakes!
We keep putting Songs on
your phone and you seem to
enjoy it!!
you told the nurse that you had
4 children (& 3 Girls and 3 Boys)

She pointed out that came to
6!
Maybe you were thinking of
Clive or John George? Who
by the way has rang me every
day asking about you. Clive
is worried too and wants to visit.
I keep showing you pictures of
people and asking you to name
them but you found that really
difficult and you told me you
didn't like it. I showed you a
picture of you skiing and asked
you if you remember skiing you
told me 'no' but said you knew
it was very important to someone
I asked if you knew who that
person was and you said well
that must be Josh!

We showed you a picture of minnie mouse and you didn't know who it was.

Since my last visit (on your birthday) I have been back at work so I have heard from Charlotte and dad about your progress.

Charlotte said you seemed to know who Annie was and you asked her if she was looking after work.

apparently Dad said roger is visiting tomorrow and you correctly identified him as your boss.

I am looking forward to visiting tomorrow to see you improvements for myself!

lots of love Hannah xxx

Wednesday 13th March

Sorry for the dodgy writing, I
broke my finger in netball...
oops!
Your progress is amazing, you
went on an exercise bike today
... amazing! You're also eating
on your own and beginning to
walk.
Today I get an A* in my English
retake... 62 marks! Highest in
my year, I know you'd be
proud.
Sally Furlong and Annie Hubb
came to see you today
apparently you were delighted
to see them.
I love you loads
Sarah xxxxxx.
        xxxxxx
        xxxxx

235

Thursday 14th March

Hi mum,
I managed to get the day off work today so that i could see you before i went off to Ireland.
I walked in and you were eating your lunch by yourself You seem to have improved so much since i last saw you on monday.
Your memory has improved a lot and you told me that Annie had been to visit you said that she told you She was looking after work and you said But she would say that even if she wasnt looking after work.

Which is true I suppose.
Grandad got the train down
to visit you and then your
boss roger came uh.
he was really nice and
was excited to get back
to work and tell everybody
how well you were doing.
They have removed the plaster
for your trachy so now
you have a big hole in your
neck.
Dad and sarah then
turned up and we wheeled
you down to day care.
Dad was telling you
that people on facebook
were asking about you
and he mentiond their
Julie Lovegrove

had said something, he
told you they were coming
to visit on monday
and you said, they are
going to travel around the
world & you said 'first stop
ME!'.
we were really impressed you
had rememberd all this.
when i left you said
'raise lots of money'.
which i assumed was in
reference to my job
as a fundraiser!
r really didn't want to leave
you as i knew it would be
a while before i could
see you again.
I love you so much, stay
strong and keep up the good work
XX XX X XX

14/3/13

looking great today! you dont
look too bad yourself Roger came
to see you and you looked
very happy to see him, you asked
him about work and he said
it is all going well and not to
worry you are getting better
every day! Love you, Josh
xxxx

17/3/13

We all visited today.
Again you have made
amazing improvements
however you desperate
to come home and are
begging for us to take
you. We want you home
but we want you to get
all the help you need so
your begging makes it
very hard especially for
Dad!

Love you mum

Cholie bean

Monday 18th March 2013

Hi mum,

You looked so strong today, not just outside but inside too! You're getting argumentitive and sarcastic which makes me laugh at times! Granny and Grandad, Di Smith and me and dad came to see you. You kept begging us to take you home which was tough but we're just doing whats best for you! You said some hilardus stuff for example "I worked my socks off on the spin bike and then realised I'd only been on it for 1 minute! A MINUTE!" Haha bless you, I'm sure you'll be back to normal in no time.

I try to keep you updated on what's happening but I often forget. Oh! The women next door is such a character, the cheeky bugger stole your cream eggs! Hahaha, doubt you would have eaten them anyway.

I can't wait for you to get home, I know you want to be here too but it shouldn't be too long.

I love you to infinity and beyond.
Sarah
xxxxxx
xxxxxx
xxxxxx

19/3/13

So I came at around
11:45 to visit Sarah the
occupational therapist
came to see me and she
said your assessment for
Sevenoaks neuro trauma
centre is on Friday
morning so Dad is
planning on being there
with you!!
Your still moaning about
being there but you
seemed to suggest that
it was the night you
didn't like there because
you said you worry to
much about things.
We won't you to come
have to but you need the

Input that they give you
in hospital and also
they say you won't be
safe out here because
you will forget you left
the hob on for example.
Di was in when I
arived you enjoyed her
company and you said
the Byrd's had seen
you earlier in the morning
I think someone else had
visited too but not sure
uno.
You had Physio today
and I got to watch
you did some Funrea;
yoga live thing tha I'm
pretty sure I couldn't do

and she had you on your
hands and knees but
your ® shoulder was
playing up and she
said she thought you
had a 'frozen' shoulder!
   Then Dad and Sarah
arrived and you managed
9 minutes on the treadmill
quite fast and then we
played catch and then
you had to throw bean-
bags into hoops and then
a little assault course
and a stroll outside up
a big hill.
   You did side steps
and balance tasks.!! AMAZING!!
   We painted your nails
and I gave you a hand

message and we watched
'one DAY' the movie
so we were soooo busy.
Then we left... nope
I lied we then went to
a shop in the hospital
and a cafe and then
we left!!
... Today was a busy
day!!!

love you madly

XXXXX

19th March 2013   Sarah

We came to see you today
but you weren't in your bed!
Turned out you were doing some
physio with Charlie and your
physio therapist. You were on
the tread mill for 5 mins!
Amazing! We then played catch
and went outside for a walk
... it was too cold!
After that we took you to
the café and we had a
drink, it was lovely.
You looked shattered when we
left you so fingers crossed
you slept through the night!

Love you SO much mum,
Sarah.,

xxxxxxxxxx

22/3/13

You got assessed today by the neuro team in Sevenoaks and it seems like the place to go you are a [crossed out] a little bit too wobbly on your feet to be accepted just yet because you will have your own bedroom.

You did loads today and seemed pretty excited about our day trip tommorow.

Love you
Charlie bean.

Xxxx X

248

23/3/13   Hannah

I have had to go
back to work for a week
so I haven't seen you since
the 13th March.
However last week (wed)
my phone pinged + I checked
my facebook page only to
find that you had commented
on a post !!!
I couldn't believe it! I rang
dad and he confirmed that
you had done it by yourself?
You commented
"needs logo" "need to jog"
"need to "plan way home"!"
"feels upset staff fentastic, its
me?"   "Dad tell please"
which seems to suggests you
don't like being in the hospital

In fact you have been telling
alot of people that you
are very upset being at the
hospital.
We would love to bring you
home but the Doc's are
strongly advising against it
I spoke to you on the
phone a few times and
the second time, I told
you I would be visiting
on Saturday and you
said your being assessed
on Friday and there
is a small chance you
will be moved which is
correct!
I was so impressed
that you had a very
good understanding of the

week,

Today we took you to Whitegate which made you very tired, but its the first time I have seen you in ages! And I can see you have came on leaps and ~~bda~~ bounds!

I cant believe how well you are doing!

27/03/13

I know this is late but things have been pretty busy and guess what? I'm ill. I have the flu or something... Sicks. Anyway, we got some great news yesterday, your coming home tomorrow (thursday) and leaving on Tuesday to go to Sevenoaks, I bet you can't wait!

I'm so excited to have you back, when you get better we have to have a party and go shopping in Bluewater like we use to.

I love you like crazy,
Sarah

xxxxxxxx
xxxxxxx